ACHIEVING IMPRESSIVE CUSTOMER SERVICE

7 Strategies for the Health Care Manager

Wendy Leebov, Gail Scott, Lolma Olson

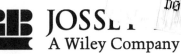

American Hospital Publishing, Inc.
An American Hospital Association Company
Chicago

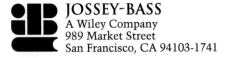

JOSSEY-BASS
A Wiley Company
989 Market Street
San Francisco, CA 94103-1741

www.josseybass.com

Jossey-Bass books and products are available through most bookstores. To contact Jossey-Bass directly, call (888) 378-2537, fax to (800) 605-2665, or visit our website at www.josseybass.com.

Substantial discounts on bulk quantities of Jossey-Bass books are available to corporations, professional associations, and other organizations. For details and discount information, contact the special sales department at Jossey-Bass.

We at Jossey-Bass strive to use the most environmentally sensitive paper stocks available to us. Our publications are printed on acid-free recycled stock whenever possible, and our paper always meets or exceeds minimum GPO and EPA requirements.

Jossey-Bass also publishes its books in a variety of electronic formats. Some content that appears in print may not be available in electronic books.

Cover design by Jeanne Calabrese

Library of Congress Cataloging-in-Publication Data

Leebov, Wendy.
    Achieving impressive customer service: 7 strategies for the health care manager / by Wendy Leebov, Gail Scott, and Lolma Olson.
       p. cm.
    Includes index.
    ISBN: 1-55648-230-2
    1. Health services administration. 2. Patient satisfaction. 3. Consumer satisfaction. I. Scott, Gail, 1946–   .
II. Olson, Lolma. III. Title.
RA971.L375   1998
362.1'068—dc21   97-51922

FIRST EDITION
PB Printing   10 9 8 7 6 5 4 3

Contents

About the Authors

Together the authors have more than 50 years of experience working inside and outside health care organizations nationally and internationally. They have developed and reinforced a customer orientation that builds the systems, skills, and spirit people need to excel at serving health care consumers.

Wendy Leebov is associate vice president of Organizational Learning and Performance Enhancement for the Albert Einstein Healthcare Network in Philadelphia, where she is responsible for organizational change and performance effectiveness strategies. Wendy was previously founder and president of the Einstein Consulting Group, a subsidiary of Albert Einstein Healthcare Network, a consulting firm specializing in helping health care organizations launch and sustain comprehensive service and quality improvement strategies. A nationally recognized speaker, author, and consultant, Wendy has worked with health care organizations nationwide and in Japan. Wendy has her BA degree from Oberlin College and her master's and doctorate from the Harvard Graduate School of Education.

Wendy Leebov's other publications include *Service Savvy Health Care: One Goal at a Time* (with Susan Afriat and Jeanne Presha, 1998); *Service Quality Improvement: The Customer Satisfaction Strategy for Health Care* (with Gail Scott, 1994); and *The Health Care Manager's Guide to Continuous Quality Improvement* (with Clara Jean Ersoz, MD, 1991).

Gail Scott is president of Gail Scott and Associates in Meadowbrook, Pennsylvania. Gail is a nationally recognized consultant and speaker on organizational change strategies, team building, leadership development, and service improvement. Formerly, Gail was director of consulting practice and president for the Einstein Consulting Group in Philadelphia. For more than 20 years, she has worked with more than 500 health care clients in the United States and beyond. A recognized author, Gail has coauthored several books with Wendy Leebov: *Service Quality Improvement: The Customer Satisfaction Strategy for Health Care; Healthcare Managers in Transition: Shifting Roles and Changing Organizations*; and (also with Michael Vergare) *Patient Satisfaction: A Guide to Practice Enhancement*. Gail is on the faculty of the American College of Healthcare Executives. She received her BA and MA degrees from Beaver College in Pennsylvania.

Lolma Olson is president of Sage Consulting, specializing in organizational transformation and service improvement. Lolma has over 25 years of experience in organization development and patient/customer relations. She served as a consultant in change management, customer relations, creating healing environments in health care settings, team building, and negotiation and conflict resolution for medical centers, outpatient clinics, and associated health care settings. Formerly she was president of the California Patient Relations Association and director on the board of the Society for Healthcare Consumers (formerly the National Society for Patient Representation and Consumer Affairs). Lolma has a master's certificate in organizational development from the California Institute of Integral Studies in San Francisco.

Acknowledgments

We thank our clients and colleagues over the years who, because of their determination to improve service quality for the sake of health care consumers, helped us experiment, learn, and grow. Special thanks also to our friends who supported us throughout the writing process.

Wendy Leebov extends heartfelt appreciation to Blanche Labovitz, Florence and Mike Leebov, Jewel Hyland, Nikki Gollub, Linda Goldston, Mary Ellen Barnett, Julie Scenna Fitzgibbons, Sharon Bergen, Jeanne Presha, Susan Afriat, Lynne Kornblatt, Audrey Jadczak, Ora Douglass, and everyone in the Albert Einstein Healthcare Network for being her best cheerleaders, teachers, and inspiration.

Gail Scott would like to thank Tom Quinlan, always; her partners and role models, Lynda Rothman, Amy Unrath, Diane Boynton, Carolyn Kettenacker, Steve Mandle, Mary Plummer, Warren Kessler, Pam Maiolatesi, Carol Wolff, Pat Mathews, Laura Blickensdorfer; the talented folks at Key Management Strategies; and the wonderful clients that she has been privileged to work with and learn from over the years.

Lolma Olson gives special thanks to Beth Reed, Barry Bastian, Linda Silver, and all the clients she works with who care so much about people and give so much of themselves in so many incredible, healing ways.

Introduction

After years of focusing on cost, trailblazing health care organizations are recognizing that impressive customer service will set them apart. They recognize the need not only to satisfy, but to *impress* their customers, to dazzle them, in order to win their loyalty. After all, it's customer loyalty that will translate into customer retention for the future. As our health care system changes, it's becoming clear that choice among providers will continue to be preserved. Patients and other customers will maintain the power to say no to poor and even adequate service; they'll insist on giving their business to the providers that excel on service dimensions. Health care providers of all sizes and shapes will embrace the need to compete on service dimensions or risk losing business to the provider down the street.

The Rocky Path to Service Improvement

Despite the fact that many organizations have recognized the importance of great customer service to maintaining their competitive position, service improvement is rarely a systemwide priority. Why is this?

- Health care leaders in large and small organizations are swamped. They're considering or executing mergers, acquisitions, affiliations, and new ventures. They are consumed by changing payment mechanisms and shifts to managed care. Although they recognize the competitive benefits of impressive service, it's hard to concentrate on it.

- Some health care leaders, especially those embroiled in new organizational configurations, question the sense of initiating massive internal change processes. They yearn for high levels of satisfaction and loyalty from all of their customers, yet they recognize the difficult challenge of making this happen organizationwide. If it were easy, it might be different.
- In some organizations, service line managers, heads of ambulatory care settings, medical practice administrators, and the like have been told by higher-ups to improve service but lack the resources or guidelines for doing so.

Although leaders of health care organizations large and small believe that impressive service is critical for mission fulfillment and competitive success, they want managers to take the bull by the horns and, with a high degree of autonomy, lead service improvement initiatives. The individual manager is the only one close enough to frontline service delivery. He or she is close enough to the team to keep the approach simple and manageable, and close enough to customers to listen and address their needs and concerns in a timely fashion. But individual managers don't necessarily have the wherewithal to improve the service aspects of their business. Often, too much is expected of them already. In large or multilayered organizations, many feel sandwiched between senior management, staff and physicians, and customers, and often feel alone in their role. In small services, many feel alone or unsure how to focus staff on service when people have diverse roles and lots of pressure.

The Purpose of This Book

Achieving Impressive Customer Service has two main purposes:

1. We aim to describe in detail a rich array of simple, doable strategies that, one at a time or in tandem, will help you make significant improvements in service and customer satisfaction.
2. We intend to give the people responsible for a service the ability to move forward autonomously with easy-to-use strategies.

The Seven Strategies

So, without further ado, here are the strategies we concentrate on in this book:

Strategy 1:	Hire service savvy people.
Strategy 2:	Establish high standards of customer service.
Strategy 3:	Help staff hear the voice of the customer.
Strategy 4:	Remove barriers so staff can serve customers.
Strategy 5:	Reduce anxiety to increase satisfaction.
Strategy 6:	Help staff cope better in a stressful atmosphere.
Strategy 7:	Maintain your focus on service.

Because your services differ and you have so many priorities, we've seen to it that these strategies accomplish the following:

- *Offer simple ways to spark service improvement.* We selected the strategies included here on the domino principle that any strategy included should trigger a domino effect or ripple into other positive effects on service and customer satisfaction.
- *Give you options.* You can pick and choose strategies that make sense for you in your new roles and organizational configurations.
- *Complement one another.* If you and other managers from your organization choose to institute different strategies, it will work perfectly well because your efforts will complement yet be independent of each other.
- *Help you follow through on previous service and quality improvement strategies.* In big organizations, administrators can advise you to pick any one approach that meets your service's particular needs, and trigger constructive follow-up activity by managers and work teams responsible for specific areas. You can add depth to previous service strategies without adding complexity.
- *Can be used autonomously.* You can jump in without waiting for leadership or approval by higher-ups. These strategies are within the individual manager's authority and span of influence.
- *Engage your staff's energy and motivation.* You can't improve service alone because it's too much work. You need to work with staff because staff are key. They deliver the service and they need to feel responsibility and pride in making it work.
- *Show you ways to diagnose and act.* This book helps you to diagnose what you need and provides the concrete tools and alternative tools to address these needs.

Can Me, Myself, and I Improve Our Service?

Absolutely, but not alone. If you have a tendency to feel powerless in the face of a big organization of which your service is only a tiny part, you can get relief here. You have tremendous ability to make a difference in the quality of customer service and therefore to attract more customers to your services in the future. If you're motivated to exercise your power, you'll collect allies along the way.

You can make a difference in service quality despite the following obstacles:

- Even if your plate is overloaded and your staff feel overwhelmed and very, very busy
- Even if your parent organization isn't focusing on service as a priority
- Even if previous efforts to improve service have fizzled
- Even if no experts or higher-ups are available to help you

You just have to take the lead and engage your staff.

What If Your Plate Is Overloaded and Your Staff Feel Overwhelmed and Very, Very Busy?

That may be, but can you dare to make efforts to better satisfy customers a secondary concern by waiting for a time when you and your staff get less busy? The challenge is to pursue service improvements *in bite-sized pieces*. With that approach, you'll build staff confidence in the effort because they'll see the payoffs. You don't have to institute complex, multifaceted strategies to make a difference.

What If Your Parent Organization Isn't Focusing on Service as a Priority?

If you're part of a bigger organization, the energy and attention of higher-ups might be consumed by other priorities. But that doesn't mean you can't focus on internal service improvement. You're closer to the front line of service delivery. You oversee the systems and performance that affect customers directly. You are in the best possible position to make significant improvements by engaging your staff in the process. The fact is, in a service, there's a lot you can change within your span of influence, and that's where we'll help you focus your energy.

What if Previous Efforts to Improve Service Have Fizzled?

Perhaps your organization has implemented a service and/or quality improvement strategy that fizzled in the past. Maybe it fizzled because people stopped paying attention, or they felt successful and didn't follow up, or became distracted and didn't follow up, or because it was too hard to manage. Or perhaps they gave up because the results were disappointing when compared to the investment of time and energy. All of that may be. But the fact is, the need to satisfy customers didn't fizzle. To help your services thrive, you need to find manageable approaches to effective service—approaches that don't depend on loads of other people or on an organization-wide grand plan.

What if No One Is Available to Help You?

There's a lot you can do without the involvement of people beyond your service—if you harness the energies of your staff and don't try to do too much at once. Without your staff on board, your impact will indeed be limited.

You Can Take the Reins

It's within your power to improve service quality and customer satisfaction, which is crucial to meeting your service and business goals. You're probably accountable for satisfying customers whether or not you're getting any help doing it or whether or not your staff feel too busy.

What can you do? Take the reins. Institute your own approaches to improving service within your span of influence. Look at your service as one team delivering specific services, and you can greatly improve the team's quality of service.

You don't need an exhausting or an exhaustive approach. There are many manageable strategies you can use, one at a time, to engage your team in making service improvements.

The Contents

Each of the first seven chapters of this book tackles one of the strategies in detail. In chapter 1, "Hire Service Savvy People," we provide the method and tools needed to screen job applicants for competencies key to great customer service. We'll go beyond exhortations about how important this is (you already know that) and instead tell you how! After all, if you hire service stars, you don't have to coach and teach, counsel and obsess about the customer service skills you wish they had in addition to their technical skills.

You'll find options for getting your staff and your team committed to raising standards in chapter 2, "Establish High Standards of Customer Service." You'll be able to work with staff to identify important service behaviors for all staff to exhibit as well as how to make these behaviors job specific in the form of service scripts and protocols. You'll then find tools for setting measurable service standards that function as promises you make to your customers. And, finally, you'll see tools for setting service targets or specific goals that focus your standard-raising pursuits.

In chapter 3, "Help Staff Hear the Voice of the Customer," you'll find simple strategies that help staff adopt their customers' perspectives. These include strategies that channel feedback from customers directly to frontline staff; short simulations that you can conduct in order to help staff see your services through the eyes of your customers; and techniques for helping staff remember their customers' perspective in the midst of everyday work pressures.

In chapter 4, "Remove Barriers so Staff Can Serve Customers," you'll find ways to help staff reduce the frustrations they create for each other that impede service. You'll find techniques for providing clear direction and contingency plans so people know what to do when service breaks down. And you'll find techniques for questioning and modifying everyday practices so that staff have an expanded latitude to act on their customers' behalf.

Chapter 5, "Reduce Anxiety to Increase Satisfaction," gives you the step-by-step tools needed to apply a far-reaching research finding about the relationship between anxiety reduction and customer satisfaction.

Chapter 6, "Help Staff Cope Better in a Stressful Atmosphere," provides alternative approaches for refueling and reenergizing staff who feel overloaded, overwhelmed, or drained from serving numerous customers in a high-pressure environment. Techniques include how to engage staff in creating a supportive *work space*; how to develop the coping skills needed in a high-stress service environment; how to help staff *unhook* when others are losing it around them; and how to build a supportive work group.

Work overload and multiple demands compete for your staff's attention every day, making it hard for them to remember to keep their focus on service. In chapter 7, "Maintain Your Focus on Service," you'll find ways to build your service focus into everyday events and interactions. You'll also find the details of an approach to engage staff in improving high-priority service behaviors one behavior at a time. And, finally, you'll find a compendium of recognition devices that help you, team members, and customers to celebrate your team and each other for making service improvements and achieving high levels of customer satisfaction.

Finally, chapter 8, "Getting Personal," describes what it takes for you to become the driver of service improvement. Valuable tips and tools will help you decide where to start, how to select approaches right for your situation, and how to gain significant support and help to make your service improvement pursuit easier, more productive, more educational, and more personally gratifying.

The Audience

We wrote this book with the following people in mind:

- Service and product line managers in hospitals, networks, and systems
- Heads of medical practices
- Managers in managed care organizations/HMOs
- Administrative physicians
- Physicians and managers of medical practices
- Managers of outpatient, ambulatory care centers, and clinics
- Managers of ancillary services including labs, radiology
- Middle managers in acute care and support services
- Managers in long-term care facilities and home care agencies
- Every other type of health care provider

Others who can benefit because they influence and interact with health care managers include the following:

- Health care administrators who want to provide managers with the tools they need to make service improvements
- Change agents in health care responsible for helping work teams improve the quality of service and customer satisfaction

(such as patient/member relations leaders, organization development professionals, marketing professionals, and the like)

- Consultants and marketing professionals who help service providers improve service quality and customer satisfaction
- Education, training, and organization development professionals who help health care staff strengthen their service and customer relations skills
- Faculty in health care and service-related educational programs who want to go beyond conceptual thinking and provide *practical* tools for improving service
- Drug and equipment companies and other suppliers to health care organizations who want to be perceived by their provider customers as customer oriented

Conclusion

The tools are here. They might be unfamiliar, but they aren't hard. Jump in. Try them out. Make them work, and you and your team will create and sustain a service that impresses your customers and engenders in you and your team a gratifying pride in your contributions to the all-important health care mission.

Chapter 1

• • •

Hire Service Savvy People

Do You Need to Read This Chapter?

Consider the following questions and think about how they apply to your hiring process:

- Have you made hiring mistakes and now you feel stuck with staff who have disappointing customer service behavior?
- Do you wish you had staff members who are more effective at customer service?
- Do you often find yourself thinking that people either have it or they don't when it comes to customer service? Do you brood over the difficulty of making people into something they're not?
- Do you rue the day you hired certain people for their technical skills, because now you're left with customer service horrors to manage?
- Do you fully recognize the importance of hiring people who are already inclined toward good customer service, but you just don't know how to screen for them effectively?
- Have you been conned by applicants who seem great at customer service in the job interview but who then turn out to be big disappointments once they're in the job?
- Do you wish you nipped customer service performance problems in the bud during hiring and probation since it's so much harder to terminate people later because of the requirements of your progressive discipline system, labor laws, and the like?

If you answered yes to even one of these questions, read on. You've paid a price for hiring the way you do—a price you don't have to pay. This chapter will show you how to develop and use hiring tools to identify applicants who have great customer service skills in addition to the technical competencies you seek.

Headaches and Heartache: The Price of Lamentable Hiring

When you pick people without testing them for customer service potential, you might very well end up with terrific experts on the technical aspects of the job. But, the headaches begin when the individual interacts with your patients and other customers. People who lack customer orientation and finely honed customer service skills turn customers off and away. Also, when people on your team turn off customers, others on your team (including you) need to spend time redoing the job or repairing the damage. You then have to confront the staff member who wronged the customer and handle their emotions and yours. And that's still not the end of it. You then have to keep watch to see whether the problem continues. Who has the time or emotional energy for all this? All of this is costly, time consuming, and draining to you, not to mention the fact that customers are affected; they leave your service unimpressed at best or disillusioned at worst.

When you hire service savvy staff, it's a different story. Good things befall you. You don't have to worry about what your staff member will say to the next customer and the one after. You don't have to worry that the next interaction will create problems that force you to drop everything and intervene. You can assume that staff are helping to satisfy customers and build their loyalty, which, in turn, inclines customers to return to your service in the future and recommend it to others. This is good for patients, for your service's reputation, and for business. And you will certainly sleep better.

The Problem

Most methods of hiring don't screen people very well at all. We tend to be best at finding out whether people have the technical skills and experience they need to perform those aspects of the job, although we even make mistakes there. And when it comes to screening for customer service, if we remember to do it at all, we ask questions like "What have you done before? What do you see as your greatest strengths?" and other questions that give the candidate a golden opportunity to show not their customer service skills, but their skills at selling themselves and reconstructing past reality to help them get the job. You learn hardly anything about what the candidate has really done, how they've behaved in the past, their real skill levels, and how they're likely to behave in the future.

The Solution

The answer is behavior-based screening. If you want to trust what you learn, question candidates differently and also test them right in the interview environment. Test candidates to see if they can do what they say they can do, so you can judge for yourself whether their skill level fits your needs.

More about the Wonderful Techniques of Behavior-Based Screening

Behavior-based screening is founded on two principles:

1. Past behavior is the best predictor of future behavior.
2. If you want to see whether people can do a skill, make them use the skill then and there. Then, decide for yourself.

Hiring methods based on these principles look really different from the usual hiring practices. There are two such methods:

1. Ask questions during the interview that dig for specifics about the applicant's past experiences.
2. During the interview, ask the applicant to perform tasks that require the candidate to show his or her competency.

Interview Questions

When you ask questions in an interview, ask candidates to describe in detail past situations and their specific behavior, results, and feelings in those situations. Most people can describe situations in general, even if they weren't there or weren't key players in the situation. But few people can construct detailed facts from scratch. They can't write fiction on the spot. They had to be there to be able to produce facts and details on demand about a situation. When you push for these details, you find out what they really did.

Thanks to Janine Kilty, senior vice president at the Albert Einstein Healthcare Network, here are two tips that make you effective in the interview itself when you ask behavior-based questions:

1. *Push for specifics and more specifics.* Probe for the details by asking such questions as "And exactly what happened next? And then what happened? And exactly what did you feel? And exactly what did you think? And exactly what did you do? And exactly what did the customer do then?" By probing for the details, you'll hear the story and know if it's true by the person's ability to produce the details.
2. *Push for "I" not "we."* Another trick in behavior-based interviewing is to focus the person on their individual role in the situation and push them to depart from the use of the word "we." When they say "we," say something like, "I realize you worked as part of a team in that situation and that probably explains why you're saying 'we.' But I'm very curious to know what your role was exactly. Please tell me what you did in particular—in detail." People who struggle at this point are revealing that they didn't have a significant role as an individual. They are probably talking about what other people did.

Performance Tasks

These tasks must be doable in a short period of time. You present a typical situation that calls for the competencies you seek and ask the candidate to handle the situation as best they can.

To facilitate performance tasks effectively do the following:

1. *Press the candidate to show, not tell.* Push them to show their competency by acting out the situations posed to them, instead of talking about these situations. Say, as often as you need to, "Please respond as if I am the customer and you are on staff . . . as if this is really happening here and now. Don't tell me how you would respond. Actually respond to me as if the situation is happening now."

2. *If they make it easy, you make it harder.* If the candidate handles the interaction very briefly, add elements to it. For instance, if you're playing a customer, resist what they're saying. Make it harder for them. Apply pressure and you'll learn much more about how they handle situations; you'll learn about the words they use, their ability to handle emotion and stay composed, and much more.

For interview questions about the past and for performance tasks, don't let them off the hook. Often in interviews when a candidate appears stumped and silent, the interviewer becomes uncomfortable with the silence and either withdraws the question, changes it, or gives hints. Don't! Instead say, "I realize you need time to think. I can wait. Take all the time you need." Then, the applicant has to think and respond, and you'll learn about their skills as a result.

Getting Specific

Here are five straightforward tools for selecting people great at customer service using behavior-based screening:

1. Screen frontline staff on four customer service competencies.
2. Screen managers and supervisors on the customer focus competency, described later.
3. Develop your own questions and performance tasks for other competencies you seek.
4. Set up your hiring process for better results.
5. Screen current staff using the same methods (so you can rehabilitate or rid your team of people who lack the skills you want).

The following sections discuss each of these tools in detail. When you use behavior-based screening methods well, you'll successfully select people you can trust to handle your customers with care and skill—people you won't have to brood about later.

Screen Frontline Staff on Four Customer Service Competencies

When you have an open position, this tool will help you pick people who are great at customer service. The following are four customer service competencies for frontline staff:

1. Emotional awareness and concern
2. Problem solving
3. Initiative and responsibility
4. Explaining and informing

After a careful analytical process, Susan Afriat, Jeanne Presha, and Wendy Leebov of the Albert Einstein Healthcare Network in Philadelphia pinpointed these four competencies as core customer service competencies. They are considered core competencies because they apply to so many situations. They help you handle a phone call with a customer, handle a customer complaint, meet a customer for the first time, conduct a procedure with a customer, ask questions to get information, and much more. They cut across many, many situations. These competencies characterize staff who are versatile and skilled at customer service. If these competencies ring true for your needs, select from the interview questions and performance tasks developed for the Albert Einstein Healthcare Network staff (and save yourself work).

Methods
The following subsections deal with each of the four core competencies and offer standard questions and performance tasks to screen candidates.

Competency 1: Emotional Awareness and Concern
A person who possesses this competency understands him- or herself and others; listens and hears customers' emotions, concerns, and needs; communicates in ways that connect with the customer at a human level; and doesn't focus only on the task or business at hand. The following are some key behavioral abilities:

• Reading others well, including both verbal and nonverbal behavior
• Showing empathy for customers' feelings and concerns
• Building rapport well with all kinds of people
• Remaining calm and focused on the customer in the face of stress
• Recognizing when emotions are getting in the way of dealing effectively with a customer

Here are some sample interview questions and performance tasks that can help you pinpoint emotional concern in applicants for positions in your service:

Interview Questions and Performance Tasks That Screen for Emotional Awareness and Concern

1. Observe the candidate during the meeting and greeting process. Do they instinctively behave in ways that build rapport with people? Watch for the following:
   —Friendliness: Smiling with mouth and eyes
   —Pleasant tone of voice
   —Firm handshake
   —Introduction
   —Pleasantries, such as "Nice meeting you."
   —Use of "please" and "thank you"
2. Say, "I'm going to read a few statements. Imagine that a patient approaches you in the hall and says each one. Listen to each statement and respond as if I were that patient":
   —"I've been waiting for two hours. What good is an appointment anyway!?"
   —"I've been ringing for a nurse for an hour! What's the matter with this place!!!"
   —In the elevator, someone says to you, "My doctor said I could stay in the hospital until I felt better and now they're making me leave!"
   —"They told me I could go into the doctor's office with my mother and I want to go in there!"
   —"I'm in a lot of pain—why won't you give me anything for it?"
   —"They brought my son to the emergency room and I can't find him!"
   Listen for:
   —Acknowledgment of customer's feeling
   —Accepting manner
   —Composure
   —Nonverbal expressions of concern, such as nodding, eye contact, focused attention
3. Say to the candidate, "I'm going to give you three situations and I would like you to listen for the customer's feeling. Act as if I'm the customer, and respond to me as you might in a real situation." After you read each situation, ask these two questions:
   —What do you think this patient is feeling?
   —Tell me what you would say if I were the patient.

And listen for:
—Recognition of patient's feeling; empathy
—Statement of concern/care

Situation A
Nurse: "I brought your medicine, Mr. Jones."
Mr. Jones: "I do not want it. People are always telling me to do this, do that, do this, do that! I'll take that medicine when I feel like it!"

Situation B
Patient: "Sometimes I think my family could do just as well without me. It's like I died already. They hardly ever come to see me."

Situation C
Patient: "I don't see why I had to sit here for two hours just to be seen for one minute!"

4. Say to the candidate, "Think of a time when a customer was really nasty to you." Ask the following questions:
—What happened?
—How did you feel?
—What did you say?
—What did you do?
Listen for:
—Description of situation and problem
—Patient listening
—Attempt to acknowledge customers' feelings
—Nondefensive, empathetic response
—Composure, calmness in the face of unpleasant customer
—Calm assertiveness if boundaries needed to be set to prevent abuse of staff

5. Ask the candidate to talk about their perceptions of the stresses of hospitalization on patients and their family members. Listen for the following responses and any others that show empathy on the part of the candidate.
—Patients worry about whether they'll get better.
—Patients worry that no one will care about them and that they'll be lost in the system.
—Patients are overwhelmed by language, people, results, and procedures they don't understand.
—Patients worry that they'll be left alone and forgotten.

Competency 2: Problem Solving

A problem solver identifies problems, finds common ground, and provides solutions and options that are in the best interests of both the customer and the organization. Here are some component behaviors:

- Asking questions to find out more about the problem
- Listening to customers and pinpointing problems to be solved
- Resourcefulness; generating workable options and solutions good for both customers and the organization
- Asking for help when a problem goes beyond your ability to solve it

These questions and tasks help to identify good problem solvers:

Questions and Performance Tasks That Screen for Problem Solving

1. Ask the candidate, "Describe a time when a customer spoke up about a problem with the service he or she was getting." Probe further with the following questions:
   —What exactly was the situation? What did the customer complain about?
   —What exactly was the problem from his or her point of view?
   —What exactly was the problem from your point of view?
   —How did you respond?
   —What were the options you offered the customer?
   —What happened?
   —How did you feel about the result?
   —How do you think the customer felt about the result?
   Listen for the following:
   —Clear statement of the problem
   —Offering of solutions
   —Alternatives/options for the customer
   —Resolution of the problem
2. Pose this situation: "A nurse takes medicine to Mr. Jones. Mr. Jones says, 'I do not want it. People are always telling me to do this, do that, do this, do that! I'll take that medicine when I feel like it!'" Ask the candidate these questions:
   —What's the problem here?

—Can you think of three options for handling this situation?
Listen for a clear statement of the problem and workable options.

3. Pose another situation: "A patient says, 'Sometimes I think my family could do just as well without me. It's like I died already. They hardly ever come to see me.'" Ask these questions:
   —Can you think of three options for handling this situation?
   —What are the pros and cons of each option?
   —Which option would you choose, and why?
   Listen for a clear statement of the problem and workable options.

4. Pose the following situation: "Mrs. Hart is waiting for an appointment and comes to the desk and says, 'What's taking so long? My appointment with Dr. Herman was for noon and it's 1:30 and I can only stay another half hour.' The fact is, Dr. Herman was expected but isn't there yet." Ask these questions:
   —Can you think of three options to give Mrs. Hart?
   —What are the pros and cons of each option?
   —Which option would you choose, and why?
   Again, listen for a clear statement of the problem and workable options.

Competency 3: Initiative and Responsibility

An employee with initiative and responsibility takes action to satisfy customers, makes decisions, and takes responsibility for outcomes. These are component behaviors:

- Taking personal responsibility for creating a positive experience for customers
- Greeting customers in a warm, professional manner; breaking the ice to help them feel welcome and important
- Acting quickly to meet customer needs and ease their concerns
- Following through to make things happen
- Apologizing when things go wrong for the customer even if it's not your fault

Applicants with initiative and a strong sense of responsibility will respond to questions and tasks like these:

Interview Questions and Performance Tasks That Screen for Initiative and Responsibility

1. Pose a situation such as the following: "The front desk person learned that a doctor canceled for the day. She was supposed to call patients to cancel their appointments. A patient arrives and finds out that there is no caregiver there to see her. The receptionist had called her, but she wasn't home." Ask these questions:
   —How would you handle the situation if you were the receptionist?
   —What would you say?
   Listen for the following:
   —Apology, with "I" not "we" or "they" language.
   —Taking responsibility, offering personally to help or find help or options.
2. Say to the candidate, "Many people are stressed and anxious when they come to an outpatient center for tests. What ideas do you have about how to relieve their stresses and anxieties?" Listen for the following:
   —Action-oriented ideas that place responsibility for patient comfort on staff initiative, not solely on customer.
   —Ideas that indicate flexibility and willingness to go beyond job descriptions and department boundaries
   —Creative ideas
3. Ask the candidate to describe a time on the job when he or she saw someone in need of comfort and provided it. Listen for the following:
   —Caring and empathy for the person and their situation.
   —Initiative and creativity in the action(s) taken.
   —Actions that required effort/time on the part of the employee

Competency 4: Informing and Explaining
A person good at informing and explaining communicates appropriate information in ways that are clear, understandable, and respectful. Such a person does the following:

- Fully informs the customer of what he or she is doing for them, to them, and with them
- Communicates in ways people can understand
- Checks to make sure customers understand and finds effective ways to get messages across

- Explains delays and other service problems and offers alternatives
- Communicates in a respectful way that does not patronize, confuse, or insult customers
- Anticipates what people will need to know and explains before they have to ask
- Encourages customers to ask questions

You can gauge applicants' ability to inform and explain with questions like the following:

Interview Questions and Performance Tasks That Screen for Explaining and Informing

1. Say, "Sometimes a customer needs something for their own comfort that we can't provide, or they ask us to do something that we aren't permitted to do. Can you think of a time when that happened? Tell me about it in detail." Use these follow-up questions:
   —Who was the customer?
   —What did the customer want that you couldn't provide?
   —Why couldn't you provide it?
   —What did you say to the customer?
   —What was the result?
   Listen for a tactful approach to saying no that includes the following:
   —Empathy for the person and their situation
   —A clear explanation that goes beyond "I can't, I'm not allowed . . ."
   —Realization of consequences of saying no.

2. Ask, "Can you think of a procedure you followed in your last job, one that had many steps to it? Explain it to me in detail. What was the purpose and what steps were involved?" Listen for the following:
   —Clear purpose
   —Clear explanation in sequence
   —Avoidance of unexplained jargon or abbreviations
   —Interest or effort to check to see if you understood

3. Give the applicant something to read about a service provided by your organization. Ask them to read it and then explain it to you in their own words. Listen for the following:
   —Clear explanation
   —Avoidance of jargon
   —An invitation to check their understanding or ask questions

4. Ask the candidate, "Describe a time that you had to explain something to someone who had difficulty understanding what you were talking about. What was it? Why was it hard for them to understand? What did you do about it?" Listen for the following:
—Awareness of when someone had trouble understanding
—Understanding and respect for diverse communication needs
—Ability to explain difficult procedures and information
—Effort/initiative to explain it differently in hopes of getting message across

5. Ask, "Describe a time you kept a customer waiting. When you arrived, what happened? What did they say? What did you say?" Listen for the following:
—Apology
—Clear explanation of delay
—Explanation that doesn't blame someone else

An Alternative: Screen for All Competencies at Once
As an alternative or supplement to testing for each competency separately, use more complex situations and analyze the candidate's response for indications of all four of the competencies.

Interview Questions and Performance Tasks That Screen for All Competencies at Once

1. Offer the candidate this situation. Explain this and also give it to the candidate in writing so he or she has a chance to review it and think about it more carefully.

   Mrs. Riley arrived ten minutes early for an appointment with the doctor. She was scheduled to be the first appointment of the day. While she sat, time passed and other patients started filling the empty chairs. At 9:30, Mrs. Riley still had not been called. By that time, she was fidgeting nervously and glancing often at her watch. At 9:40, impatient and uncomfortable, Mrs. Riley stood up and walked to the reception desk and said in a sarcastic tone, "I *hope* I'm not inconveniencing anyone, but I *did* have a 9 o'clock appointment that I made three weeks ago. My time is as valuable as the doctor's, and I want to know why I haven't been taken yet."

Ask the candidate these questions:

—What do you think the problem is here?

—What do you think Mrs. Riley is feeling and why?

—What could have been done to prevent this?

—Let's say staff didn't prevent it. What should the staff member say now to Mrs. Riley?

—Now let's say the staff member said, "This is a very busy service, and you can't expect your doctor to see you the minute you walk in the door. I'm sorry, but you'll have to wait until she's ready for you." What do you think of that response?

—Now let's say this staff person had a habit of alerting patients to delays before the patients ask—they step into the waiting area to update them if they think there will be a delay. If you did that, what might you say?

Listen for the following:

—Evidence of emotional awareness and concern

  –Empathy/acknowledgment of feeling/inconvenience

  –Nondefensive response

—Evidence of initiative and responsibility

  –The phrase "Thank you for speaking up."

  –Apology (for keeping person waiting and for not alerting them to the wait before they had to ask)

  –Comment that staff should have alerted patient to delay before patient had to protest

—Evidence of problem solving

  –Concrete offer to help/plan of action (offer to call and check on doctor)

  –Options (staying or rescheduling)

  –Suggestions to ease customer's impatience

—Evidence of informing and explaining

  –Candidate should provide an explanation

  –Explanation should be tactful, not reflecting on or blaming others or the customer

Here's an example of a response that meets the criteria:

Mrs. Riley, I'm really sorry I didn't let you know about the delay. I meant to do that. I know you were on time and I'm very sorry that you've been waiting so long. The fact is, Dr. Rhodes had a serious emergency this morning and is behind schedule. I'm going to call her right now and find out how much longer it will be. Then you'll have some choices. You can either wait or, if you prefer, I can reschedule you. In the meantime, would you like a magazine or coffee?

2. Here's another situation to pose to the candidate:

Evelyn Jones, Dr. Simon's appointment secretary, handles a variety of phone calls every day. Although she gets billing information from patients during their visits, she isn't the person who issues their bills. The outpatient billing department does that. On this particular morning, she answers the phone and Mrs. Garrett is on the line. Mrs. Garrett says in a loud voice, "I just received a bill for $130 for tests that usually cost $30 and I want this fixed!"

Ask these questions:
—What do you think Mrs. Garrett is feeling and why? How can you tell what she is feeling?
—Upon hearing her say this, what would you say to her?
—And what, if anything, would you do afterward?
Listen for the following:
—"Thank you for speaking up."
—Apology/taking responsibility
—Empathy/acknowledgment of feeling/frustration
—Explanation of who might be able to help
—Initiative to address problem or find person who can
Beware of responses such as the following:
—"I'm sorry but the mistake wasn't mine. The billing department wrote that bill. You'll have to talk to them about it. There's nothing I can do. Call the switchboard and ask for them."
Listen for responses like this:
—"Thank you for bringing this problem to my attention. I'm very sorry you received what looks to you like a mistaken bill. I'd like to connect you with Robin, our billing person. Would you mind letting me put you on hold while I try to locate her and explain the situation? And if she's available, I'll be able to transfer you to her and I'm sure she can help you. (After finding Robin) Mrs. Garrett, I located Robin and she'll be glad to help you. I'll transfer your call, but you might want to jot down her number in case we somehow get disconnected. Her number is 456-4625. And Mrs. Garrett, I'm sorry about this situation and thank you very much for calling."

Tips

- Because the options above are too numerous to pose to any one candidate, pick and choose among these techniques those that best fit the job you're trying to fill. If you feel uncomfortable or inexperienced presenting performance tasks and asking candidates to show, not tell, practice beforehand on a current staff member, so that you become more comfortable in that role. And give yourself a pep talk. Remind yourself that if you screen with these methods now, you will avoid many difficult employee performance problems later.

- Follow through. Once you've selected people who demonstrate customer service competencies, your job isn't over. New selectees become new employees and, as new employees, they need to be oriented well to the specific demands of their job. They need to learn about the exact situations they will need to handle and the work processes they will need to perform, manage, or complete. They need to get to know their customers and learn the context for applying their customer service competencies. Also, they need to receive periodic monitoring of their work and helpful coaching to ensure that they use the competencies they have in the appropriate situations and meet your standards.

- Build customer service into the paperwork. Make sure the employee has a job description that includes the customer service competencies and specific expectations you have of them when they serve customers. Also build the competencies and your customer service expectations into the job-specific goals or expectations section of their annual performance review form, so you don't forget to follow up then with feedback related to customer service performance.

- Orient employees to their customers and customer service responsibilities, not just to their technical tasks. Make sure they have in hand any service protocols, scripts, standards, and other evidence of workplace procedures.

- Provide customer service coaching. Assign a customer service buddy or peer coach, preferably someone attuned to your customers and systems and exemplary at customer service. Have them answer the new person's questions and keep an eye out for ways to help them learn the job quickly and perform it skill-fully. Also, make it clear whom they should go to when they aren't sure what's OK and what isn't OK to do for customers.

• Have each employee's supervisor set up a formal feedback meeting with the employee before the end of the employee's probationary period. The two can discuss the employee's performance, rejoice in evidence of positive contribution, flag problems, and give the employee a chance to meet any standards he or she is failing to meet. And raise the bar on customer service: talk about opportunities to be impressive. If the employee doesn't provide impressive customer service, set up a coaching session with a buddy to whom you explain the specific performance issues warranting attention, and require them to attend relevant training.

• At the end of probation, make a thoughtful decision . . . or pay later. Frequently, managers are busy and they don't give sufficient thought to whether or not to retain the employee at the end of the probationary period. Then the employee stays, and the manager later regrets it. The idea is to cut your losses if you made a mistake; do so during probation when it's easy instead of waiting until the employee feels permanent and must be guided through what might be a cumbersome and anxiety-provoking progressive discipline process.

Screen Managers and Supervisors on the Customer Focus Competency

The purpose of this tool is to help you pick people for management jobs who are customer oriented and exemplary in their customer service skills.

The definition of the Customer Focus competency and methods of screening for it were developed by the management role redesign team of the Albert Einstein Healthcare Network when they re-defined every leader's role in terms of eight key competencies.

The customer-focused manager demonstrates a desire to help or serve others—to identify, anticipate, and address customer/client needs and achieve customer satisfaction. Customers include patients, their families, employers, community, referral sources, and payers, as well as people internal to the organization who rely on services in order to perform their functions. The following are the behavioral components of a customer-focused manager:

- Gets firsthand customer information and uses it for service design, evaluation, and improvement
- Persists in providing the highest quality products/services and finding ways to better meet customer needs, including improving systems that affect customer satisfaction; keeps customer focus as the driver of planning and implementation
- Goes out of the way to communicate with customers in ways that meet their needs, while also earning their trust and respect
- Listens attentively and thoughtfully to customer issues and probes for underlying issues; responds with empathy and takes steps to address concerns; follows through to ensure that commitments are kept and issues resolved
- Takes personal responsibility for correcting customer service problems promptly and nondefensively to a point where the customer is satisfied
- Considers and treats as valued customers both internal and external users of services; acts to create and sustain positive long-term relationships
- Promotes centrality of customer focus with staff by instilling, reinforcing, and supporting staff's efforts to do all of the above.

Method

Use a combination of interview methods and performance tasks to determine whether the candidate has the customer-oriented skills and attitude you're looking for.

1. Start with interview questions. The following sample shows interview questions on customer focus, displayed on a form you can use as your rating form.

Ask	Listen for	Rating (5 = Great)
What is it that attracts you to this field?	• Customer orientation, especially patient care mission and desire to help others and to achieve customer satisfaction • Energy, excitement about the work/mission and contributing	1 2 3 4 5
In your last job, who did you see as your main customers? How would you characterize their main needs? What is something you did to cater to their needs? Exactly how did you evaluate your success in meeting their needs?	• Articulation of who customers are and their needs • Inclusion of both internal and external customers • Strategies to get firsthand customer information • Concrete, sound example of strategy to satisfy customer • Evidence of evaluating results of strategy and/or monitoring customer satisfaction	1 2 3 4 5
Give an example in your past experience when a customer had a strong complaint. What was it? How did you become aware of it? Specifically, what did you do about it?	• Persistence in providing high-quality service and finding better ways to do things • Actions to address current issue • Actions to prevent such situations in future • Communication with customers in ways that earn trust and respect • Refers customers to appropriate individuals and makes links to them • Takes personal responsibility for correcting problems promptly and nondefensively • Closing loop/communicating back to customer	1 2 3 4 5

Give an example of an effort you've made in the past to promote a customer focus among your staff.	• Overt steps to promote customer focus • Articulation of importance of customer focus • Articulation of customers and their needs • Clarity about behavior that demonstrates customer orientation	1 2 3 4 5
Give an example of something proactive you did in your work to better address customer needs and increase their satisfaction. What was the situation? What did you do? What did this involve? What were the results? How did you know?	How need was identified: • Listening to customer • Ability to take prompt action • Proactive • How it was communicated to others • Ease of answering the question	1 2 3 4 5

Overall Comments:

2. Proceed to use performance tasks that give you a chance to see customer focus in action. Ask candidates if they are willing to complete a series of tasks before the interview situation. Set up a time and have them complete these ahead of time, preparing their responses in writing or by talking into a tape recorder. Or, if that seems difficult, reenact these situations within the interview itself, still requiring candidates to complete the tasks, not talk about *how* they would do so.

Performance Task A: Video Attitude Problem

Show on video an attitude problem. For instance, a doctor asks a clerk to locate some information. She slowly gets up, drags herself over to a pile of papers, looks for it briefly, and gets distracted into a conversation with another staff member until the doctor harrumphs. She finally saunters back with the information and slaps it in front of the doctor.

Ask the candidate to plan for five minutes and then begin to conduct a coaching or discipline discussion based on what they saw. After they've done this, express to them three examples of employee resistance to being coached on this: for example, (1) I was *swamped* that day and had a workload that wasn't fair! (2) It was not my responsibility to handle this situation. (3) I do my job day in and day out. I can't believe you're focusing on this little tidbit of behavior when I just slipped. Who's perfect, after all?

Listen and look for the following:

- Behavioral description of attitude problem
- Clear explanation of why behaviors are inappropriate with customers; consequences for customer and organization
- Appropriate understanding of employee resistance points; sensitivity to employee resistance
- Appropriate responses to employee resistance that keep focus on importance of customer service and satisfaction

Performance Task B: Priorities Situation

Tell the candidate, "You're a manager. Four situations arise at once. You get a phone call from the CEO with a request to call back. You have a message from a doctor marked urgent that asks for your help in getting a patient a bed. A patient's family member is complaining about the care his or her loved one is receiving and wants your help. Your budget is due at 3 P.M. and you need at least two more hours to work on it. How would you handle these competing priorities?" Listen and look for the following:

- Customer focus: Articulation of customers and why they're important, including patient's family member and physician, and, secondarily, supervisor and CEO
- Ability to prioritize with sound rationale, including an initial focus on the patient's family member as most important
- Ability to delegate
- Resourcefulness
- Use of time under pressure
- Showing concern about *all* customers

Performance Task C: Customer Complaint Situation

Describe this situation to the candidate: "You are walking through the halls of a hospital and a person in street clothes stops you and says in a very loud voice, 'Do you work here? My daughter's here for a procedure and they called and asked me to come to pick her up. I can't find her and I've been where they told me to go. This place is awful. We can't ever get what we need when we come here! Now, what am I supposed to do?'" Ask the candidate to handle the situation as if it were happening here and now. Look for the following:

- Empathy
- Stated intention to help
- Introducing self and role as manager
- Asking person to step out of earshot of others
- Listening
- Intervening appropriately (by self or seeking others)
- Follow-through
- Sensitivity to present problem and past experience, not just present problem

Performance Task D: Complaint Letter Situation

Provide candidate with a complaint letter received by your service. Ask them to take 10 minutes to write a letter to the customer responding to this complaint. When you evaluate their response later, look for the following:

- Empathy
- Acknowledgment of feeling
- Apology that people were upset, if appropriate
- Taking responsibility
- Clear actions to be taken
- Clear explanation
- Possible options
- Appreciation for having spoken up
- Readability, organization

Performance Task E: Visitor Situation

Pose this scenario to your candidate: "You're walking down the hall. You notice that a woman coming toward you is crying and appears distraught and frustrated. Would you do or say anything or let her pass?"

If applicant says anything, follow up with, "I'm looking for the complaint department. You should see what they're doing to my mother!" and ask them, "What would you say? Pretend I'm this person and handle me as you think you would."

Look for the following:

- Empathy expressed
- Apology for having bad experience
- Taking personal responsibility
- Questions to pinpoint problem
- Initiative to follow up or find person who can help

Performance Task F: Internal Customer Situation

Ask, "One of your employees comes to you with many complaints about her work overload. This employee complains further that the job is changing and is now very different than what you led her to believe when you hired her. She is upset because she feels it's unfair to change what's in the job. How do you respond?" Listen for whether the person does the following:

- Demonstrates empathy for other's feelings and concerns
- Recognizes the impact of behavior on others
- Shows composure
- Listens patiently and asks questions to better understand
- Responds in a respectful, nondefensive manner
- Can accurately project what various people are likely to do across a variety of situations

Tips

- You don't need to use all of these situations. Pick those that best reflect the demands on managers in your service.
- These questions and tasks help you select customer-oriented people for management roles. If you pick well, you can expect a

customer focus on the part of staff because of the power you and other leaders have to set the standards in your service.

Develop Your Own Questions and Performance Tasks

The purpose of this tool is to help you figure out which competencies you seek and to develop performance-based methods that screen candidates on these job-specific competencies.

Method
Use this three-step process for figuring out what kinds of performance tasks will help you determine whether candidates have the competencies you seek.

1. Create a vision for the job.
2. Translate the vision into core competencies.
3. Develop methods for screening candidates on these competencies, including questions and performance tasks.

The following subsections discuss each step in turn and offer strategies to help you accomplish them.

Step 1: Create a Vision for the Job
To hire people with the customer service skills you want, first crystallize what these key skills are. Develop a vision of the job. Picture the job and the customers it serves, and picture staff in that job functioning at full tilt and optimal effectiveness. Start by looking at the job and getting explicit about the customer service opportunities in it, and then develop a customer service vision for the job. If you skip this step, there is a danger of overemphasizing the technical/ business aspects of the job and underplaying the customer service demands of it.

Here's a strategy for holding a customer service vision meeting with your staff. It will help you and others picture the customer service interactions and opportunities in the job you're about to fill, so you can (in step 2) pinpoint the competencies you need in candidates for the job.

Strategy: Team Meeting Format to Create a Customer Service Vision for the Job

Method

Convene a team with a stake in hiring great people for the job at hand. If there are currently other staff members holding the same job (if it's not a one-of-a-kind job), include people in that job along with others who interact with the people in the job.

With you or someone else as facilitator, ask the group to complete this chart together for each customer group served by people in this job:

Job Title _____

Customer Group _____

Main Technical/ Business Tasks at Hand	Main Customer Service Needs during Tasks	Behavior Needed to Satisfy Customer Needs	Behaviors and Opportunities That Would Impress Customer

Here's an example of a completed form:

Job Title: Billing Clerk

Customer Group: Patients in Outpatient Service

Main Technical/ Business Tasks at Hand	Main Customer Service Needs during Tasks	Behavior Needed to Satisfy Customer Needs	Behaviors and Opportunities That Would Impress Customer
Get insurance info and record in computer	• Rapport during questions • Confidentiality • Patience • Speed	• Smiles, makes eye contact • Listens to answers • Grasps customer's answers first time • Speaks so others can't hear • Speedy, efficient data entry	• Uses customer's name often • Hears answers first time • Checks for understanding • Explains why questions are important • Thanks customer for patience • Asks, "Any questions at this point?" and follows up

With the tasks spelled out and the customer service behaviors identified, engage the same group in identifying key elements or themes and crystallizing a short vision statement for the customer service aspects of the job. This worksheet might help:

Job:

Customer Service Vision for the Job:

People in this position need to contribute to customer satisfaction and loyalty by

-

-

-

-

This step can be quick, taking 30 minutes in a special meeting or existing staff meeting. By involving staff, you not only raise their awareness of what's needed by customers in this open job, but you also sharpen their customer service thinking in general, with spin-offs for their own jobs.

Encourage staff to take this seriously instead of letting people treat it as obvious or as an unnecessary exercise. It is not obvious and needs to be articulated.

Above all, create a customer service vision for the job that reflects a stretch—one that describes a star performer, not an adequate one. The point is that the open job requires star performance, and if you don't find a star, you won't hire.

Step 2: Translate the Vision into Core Competencies

Now that you have a customer service vision for the job, pinpoint more clearly the competencies you need in candidates to be sure they have the capability of fulfilling this vision once they're on the job. Use the following strategy to make the vision concrete by translating it into key customer service competencies required for people in the job.

Strategy: Translating Your Customer Service Vision into Key Competencies

Method

With the same team, ask team members to identify the key skills that a staff member needs in order to fulfill the vision for the job. Narrow these down into the vital few competencies that will have the greatest positive impact on customers. Competencies can be skills (for example, problem solving) or traits (for example, warmth) because both can be defined in behavioral terms.

Customer Service Vision for Job:

The Absolute Most Important Customer Service Competencies Needed to Fulfill This Vision

1.

2.

3.

4.

Here's the result of applying this process step to a billing clerk job:

Customer Service Vision for Billing Clerk

Billing clerks in our service need to contribute to customer satisfaction and loyalty by

- Building positive rapport and connecting to the customer at a
  human level while doing the business at hand
- Explaining why as they ask for information
- Listening well in an atmosphere of privacy
- Inviting and addressing questions and concerns fully and patiently

The Absolute Most Important Customer Service Competencies
Needed to Fulfill This Vision

1. Rapport building
2. Listening
3. Explaining

This step is based on the principle that if you don't know exactly
what you're looking for, it's going to be very hard to find it. Don't
skip this step. The more specific you get in your target competencies, the better your ultimate hiring decision.

*Step 3: Develop and Select Methods for Screening Candidates
on These Competencies*
Now that you have defined the competencies you seek in specific
terms and are ready to develop screening methods, this first strategy
will help you to prepare interview questions so interviewers can ask
effective questions designed to screen for the competencies you seek.

Strategy A: Aid to Developing Effective Interview Questions

Method

1. Ask candidates to describe in painstaking detail times they used
   the competencies your team identified as key to the open position.
   This question format works: "I'd like you to tell me in detail about a
   time when you engaged in [name the competency]."

—What was the situation?

—Can you tell me exactly how you engaged in [competency] in that situation?

—And what happened? What were the results?

2. Prepare a list of questions associated with the competencies you identified. Type them up so interviewers have the questions, the rating criteria, and what to listen for with each answer. Here's a format that works:

Customer Service Competencies for Billing Clerk: Interviewer Rating Sheet

Vision: Billing clerks in our service need to contribute to customer satisfaction and loyalty by doing the following:

- Building positive rapport and connecting to the customer at a human level while doing the business at hand
- Explaining why as they ask for information
- Listening well in an atmosphere of privacy
- Inviting and addressing questions and concerns fully and patiently

Ask	Listen/Watch for	Rating (5 = Great)
For rapport building: I'd like you to tell me in detail about a time when you established rapport with a customer even though it wasn't easy. Who was the customer? What was the situation? Can you tell me exactly how you built rapport in that situation? And what happened? What were the results?	• Mention of smiling • Eye contact • Use of customer name • Small talk to ease anxiety	1 2 3 4 5

For listening: I'd like you to tell me in detail about a time when you had to get information from a customer and you listened well to them. Who was the customer? What did you need to find out from them? How did you get the information? Can you tell me exactly how you listened? And what happened? What were the results? How could you tell if you were effectively listening to the customer?	• Explanation of information needed from customers • Description of listening behavior (verbal and nonverbal) • Reference to customers' needs when judging effectiveness, not just staff person's own information needs	1 2 3 4 5
For explaining: What's an example in your past experience when you had to explain something complicated to a customer? What was your purpose? What was it? How did you explain it? How did you know if the customer understood?	• Ability to describe components of complex explanation • Ability to describe purpose of that explanation (nonbureaucratic reason) • Ease describing method of checking for understanding—that rings true	1 2 3 4 5

By taking the time to chart your questions, you and other screeners are more likely to ask focused questions and to know what to look for as the interview proceeds.

This next tool involves performance tasks. With performance tasks, you require candidates to demonstrate their skills during the interview. You see them in action.

Strategy B: Aid to Developing Effective Performance Tasks

Method

1. To develop performance tasks, identify actual situations that require use of each key competency or several of them at once.
2. Enact the situation in the interview environment, asking the candidate to handle it directly, not to discuss how they would handle it.

Examples for the Billing Clerk Opening

To test rapport building, say this scenario to your candidate: "Imagine I am a patient, walking up to you for the first time, after the receptionist directed me to go and give you information. I'd like you to run me through what you would do in that situation. I'll be the patient and you be you and do what you would do."

Situation 1: Imagine that you are a registration clerk. I am a customer who enters your work area and walks up to you. Greet me as you would a real customer. Let me get up and do this like a customer would, and you do what you would do. (Go out the door, enter, and walk up to the candidate, stopping in front of them.) Say, "Good morning. I need to give you my insurance information." Take out your insurance card and hand it to the clerk (applicant).

Watch the candidate's greeting behavior for rapport-building competency. (Does candidate give warm hello, make eye contact, ask you to sit down, introduce him- or herself, ask your name, and thank you for stopping by?)

Situation 2: Ask the candidate to describe a situation in which they asked a customer for information and also explained something to the customer.

After the candidate defines the situation, ask them to do this with you as customer, asking questions and explaining whatever was necessary to the customer.

Interview, listen, and watch for evidence of the billing clerk competencies of rapport building, listening, and explaining.

- Effective greeting (smiling, hello, use of name, eye contact)
- Explanation of the purpose of questions
- Explanation of questions to be clear and open
- Nonverbal listening behavior (eye contact, nodding, uh-hums)
- Verbal listening behavior (for example, "yes," "I see," paraphrasing, and repeating back what customer said to confirm understanding of it)

3. Use this worksheet to help your team develop performance tasks that generate evidence of the candidate's ability to demonstrate the competencies in lifelike situations.

Competency _____		
Situations in job when competency is needed	Performance task doable in interview environment that re-creates this situation	Rating criteria: What interviewer should listen/watch for
1.		• • •
2.		• • •
3.		• • •

Tips

- If people have trouble coming up with situations, ask them to brainstorm situations they handle every day that call for each competency. From this list, you'll find good enactable situations.
- Test these tasks: Before settling on the situations, have people on your team try them out to make sure the instructions are clear. Make sure the situations are concrete enough to be usable in the interview environment, and that skilled staff exhibit the key behaviors in the heat of the performance task.

 ## Set Up Your Hiring Process for Better Results

Now that you've used the three-step process to develop interview questions and performance tasks to test for other customer service competencies, it's time to apply them to your hiring process. Depending on the size and scope of your service, involve more than one person in the hiring process. In services where staff interact with people from other services, involve a hiring team of people who share a stake in the selection decision. It also pays to involve staff who will be close coworkers of the new employees.

Method

Create instructions for the hiring process. Offer these guidelines to the person responsible for convening a hiring team:

- For each competency, assign a different question to each interviewer, so that different interviewers won't ask the same questions. Pick those questions most appropriate to the position for which you are hiring.
- Ask people to take notes and assign a rating for each question, so different interviewers can compare notes later, focusing on one competency at a time.

To interviewers/members of the hiring team offer these suggestions:

- Early in the interview, tell the applicant, "I hope you don't mind if I take notes. I want to be sure to remember everything you say."
- In interviews with candidates, interviewers should *not* talk up front about the customer service focus in your organization or service. This will clue in the applicant to talk about a commitment to customers, even when they don't spontaneously have such a commitment.
- Ask the applicant the question you're assigned to ask (to avoid redundancy from interviewer to interviewer). The coordinator of the hiring team should have circled your assigned question on the question sheets. If not, ask them to do so.
- Listen for answers that reflect skill in the behaviors listed in the "Listen for" column.
- During the interview, take notes and write comments in the column next to the question that you asked. This will remind you of what the applicant said.
- After the interview, write in your rating for that question using a scale from 1 to 5, with 5 meaning "great."

Tip

- By involving others in the process, you benefit from multiple perspectives, you increase your own confidence in your selections, and you also develop a shared stake in the success of your new hires.

Screen Current Staff Using the Same Methods

When picturing a more systematic process for selecting customer service stars, some people lament the fact that they didn't use such a process with people who currently comprise their workforce. It's not too late. You have three options:

1. Create new jobs for current staff.
2. Do mandatory competency testing on customer service.
3. Do both.

Option 1: Create New Jobs for Current Staff

Make explicit the customer service competencies in an employee's job, document these, and communicate them to the employee, saying that because of the newly explicit expectations, the job is, in effect, a new job.

- Offer employees the chance to go through a confidential assessment process on the customer service competencies (using the same screening questions and performance tasks outlined for screening new candidates).
- Offer training in the competencies for those who know they need to improve or those who discover they need to improve once they receive their results from the assessment process.
- Emphasize (and reinforce in writing) that whether employees opt to go through the developmental assessment process or not, they will, by a certain date, be held accountable for meeting the newly explicit customer service expectations.

A variation of this option can be used if you're starting up a new service that is absorbing staff from merged or phased-out services, or to upgrade the standards of existing services. Here's how such a process might look:

Strategy: How to Institute Impressive Customer Service as a New Job Requirement

1. Communicate newly explicit customer service expectations.
   —Develop new job descriptions with explicit expectations.
   —Communicate clearly the importance/vision for customer service and the specific service expectations.
2. Conduct customer service competency assessment up front for every staff person in a customer service job to identify training needs (not to screen people out of job).
3. Provide training:
   —Hold a customer service orientation/basic refresher (for *all* service staff, including clinical).
   —People who don't pass assessment also must do the following:
     –Attend Communicating with Style (a program using videotaping, personal feedback, and help from coach).
     –Be assigned service coach/buddy for on-the-job support.
     –Attend a customer service module from training curriculum.
4. Accountability
   —New to job: After adjustment time to job (for example, four weeks), do a formal review with employee and discuss whether the employee meets the customer service expectations fully. If not, provide coaching and progressive discipline process, ending in termination if necessary.
   —Ongoing: If customer service performance problems pop up after that, use progressive discipline process.
5. Customer feedback: Tailor quantitative survey and/or focus groups to include questions pertinent to staff behavior, with feedback loop that brings results to staff to spark ongoing improvement.
6. Supervisors as coaches: Those who supervise staff use monthly observations and coaching to monitor staff on customer service performance. Use a checklist made out of the customer service competencies list.
7. Ongoing skill building: Provide periodic customer service skill-building workshops tailored to ongoing needs.

This option is far better than just increasing the frequency with which you address customer service issues when talking with staff. This option makes it very clear to staff that it's a new day with new job expectations.

Option 2: Do Mandatory Competency Testing on Customer Service

Institute customer service competencies into your mandatory competency testing system if you have one. The Joint Commission for the Accreditation of Healthcare Organizations and many other regulatory review bodies require mandatory competencies with annual evidence of employee conformance. Usually, the mandatory competencies include job-specific technical skills (like blood draws, use of certain equipment, passing of safety test, CPR, and many, many more). The fact is, while some competencies *must* be tested for annually, there's no law against building competencies you value into the same system. Do this with customer service competencies.

Method

1. Define in behavioral terms the customer service competencies you want.
2. Develop assessment methods.
3. Decide which employees must show evidence of which competencies and how often. For instance, establish four customer service competencies and their associated assessment processes. Then, require that every employee demonstrate one competency per quarter by passing the appropriate test. Specify how long employees have to take and retake the test before they are terminated for failure to satisfy the competency requirement.
4. Communicate the new requirements and the methods and schedule for assessment.
5. Give people initial training opportunities to prepare for the assessment process.
6. Institute the quarterly assessment process and follow through with it.

Tip

• If you have a union environment, talk with your labor relations specialist and work out a strategy for securing union help in selecting the appropriate approach for your setting and enlisting their support.

Repercussions of Competency Testing

Do you dare get rid of people who don't take the tests and/or don't pass them? The fact is, current employees can challenge your tests in court. That's why it's better to counsel people on their performance on the job than it is to use tests as a basis for terminating their employment. If you're serious about customer service excellence being a job requirement, then use this process to bring everyone up to standards or terminate their employment. This process says to employees, "We really mean it about customer service being serious business here. We will help you fulfill very high standards that will set us apart in the eyes of our customers and do us all proud. And, for those who can't cut it (because they don't take the tests or pass them after several chances to do so), you will need to find another workplace that places a lesser value on this critical aspect of performance."

Yes, but . . .

Do all of these hiring tools and strategies reflect a radical approach? This approach does defy many managers' sensibilities. And yes, this reflects a radical approach, because so few health care organizations have ever gone beyond the emphasis on technical expertise to get serious about expecting customer service excellence from staff. People back away from it for a whole host of reasons.

Here's what some managers say and what we say in response:

Yes, but Who Has Time?

Managers tell us, "But there's so much development involved in creating competencies customized to the job and developing assessment methods. Who has time?" If you don't, then try using the generic competencies and assessment devices presented here. You'll be surprised at how well they work. And you can modify them in minor ways if you want them to have a customized feel.

Yes, but Isn't This Process Time-Consuming and Tedious?

It is definitely time-consuming to screen candidates thoroughly for positions. But it is much more time-consuming to make poor hiring decisions and pick up the pieces later. When you hire right, you have people who support your service, satisfy your customers, and make less, not more, work for you. Why not spend your energy on a hiring squad, not a firing squad?

Yes, but Won't We Deter Good Candidates?

Managers worry that if they test people, they will lose possible candidates who resent the up-front tests. However, it's all in how you frame it. Tell people you place a great value on customer service skills and ask all candidates to complete a series of customer service screening methods so you can make sure candidates have the skills you're looking for. If candidates resent this, are you sure this resentment isn't a statement about the value they place on customer service and their willingness to join a team where the customer is the driver of expectations? By backing off from systematic screening for customer service, you're in effect saying, "It's not critical. We'll chance it."

Yes, but Won't New Staff Become Disaffected if Others Aren't Service Savvy?

This is a genuine concern. New employees will become instantly disaffected if a manager screened them for customer service competencies that others don't display. So, admit to new employees that you are upgrading the standards and are therefore screening new people more carefully than ever. Tell them you plan to raise the standards for all current employees. Otherwise, you'll hire people capable of customer service excellence who won't necessarily exceed your current operating standards, especially if they see others with mediocre service skills receiving paychecks and positive performance reviews anyway.

Conclusion

Your stated commitment to customer service will be seen as lip service unless it truly isn't. Make it real by building into your hiring process interview questions and performance tasks that enable you to see people's customer service competencies and attitudes toward customers. It's an up-front investment that promises tremendous future gains.

Chapter 2

• • •

Establish High Standards
of Customer Service

Do You Need to Read This Chapter?

Ask yourself the following questions:

- Does your service have standards so clear that staff serve customers in a consistent fashion?
- Do your customers rate your staff as impressive on satisfaction surveys?
- Do you have service standards that clearly tell staff what's expected of them when serving their customers?
- Do you have job descriptions and a performance appraisal process that focus staff on how they're supposed to be serving their customers?
- Are you spending very little time responding to customer complaints—complaints that you think should never have reached your ears?
- Do you sleep well at night because your staff members receive compliments from customers about the way they've been treated?
- When you think of customer service, do you have a hard time thinking of even one problem employee?
- Do your boss or other managers recognize your service and staff for outstanding customer service performance?
- Can you honestly say you've received no complaint letters in the last month in which customers threatened to switch providers because of some dissatisfaction with your services?

- Is your staff able to focus their time on giving real care and service because complaining customers do not plague them?

If you answered yes to these questions, skip this chapter and celebrate, because you have cracked the accountability nut! If, like the rest of us, you said no to at least a few of these questions, read on.

This chapter addresses that old saw—accountability. Accountability for customer service is driven by clarity about what customers want and a strong sense of responsibility and dedication to providing it. Accountability is about having high standards and living up to them.

With customer service accountability, each team member takes responsibility and follows specific guidelines for at least satisfying and, better yet, impressing both their internal and external customers with the service they extend to them.

Rationale

Let's get two benefits of having high customer service expectations and standards out of the way. First of all, accrediting agencies (that is, the Joint Commission for the Accreditation of Healthcare Organizations, state auditors, and the like) want to see that you have them, so you should. If you not only have them but also find ways to help your staff live up to them, the benefits are much more satisfying to everyone.

It's also good to have high standards for the sake of your business goals. If customers aren't happy with your service, they'll take their business to the service down the street. That's not good for your business or for your job security, and it doesn't engender pride in your work.

When your service has high standards and you insist upon them, staff end up proud of themselves and their services. They do right by their customers and they feel better about their work. When you make high standards happen, customers and coworkers alike count on you. They know they can depend on your services and your team, and they respect you for it.

One more thing. If you involve staff in setting the standards (instead of imposing your standards on them), they'll appreciate it and might even be inspired by, instead of resentful of, those standards. They'll own the standards and be more likely to live up to them.

Standard Setting: Easier Said Than Done

But setting standards is hard.

- It takes time. There's no doubt about it and no way around it. It takes time to think through how your team should behave in different service situations. It takes time to involve staff in the decision process. It takes time to find out from your customers if your standards are on target. And it takes time to help your team embrace the resulting vision of excellent service that your standards establish. *But,* and this is a big *but,* it also takes a lot of time to not have standards. It's just time spent differently. When you don't have standards, you spend time stewing over unsatisfactory behavior, coaching employees who are not meeting your expectations, and handling complaining customers. By setting standards, you spend considerable time up front but save much more time down the road.
- Behaviors are hard to describe. Individual staff see things differently, so it's tricky to find a common language that everyone understands about how they should and shouldn't behave with customers.
- It's hard to be objective when we're talking about behaviors. Because people have different experiences with standards and with service, it's challenging to find common ground and agreement about what good and excellent service look like.
- The language is confusing. People get caught up in "What is a standard?" and "What is the difference between a standard and an expectation?" The language related to standards is indeed confusing. People use different words to mean the same things, and the same words to mean different things. Although it might not really matter in the long run, you need to make sure you define your terms within your own group.

Getting Clear on the Definitions

To avoid creating confusion in this chapter, the following glossary shows how we define the key terms related to accountability.

Glossary of Terms

Expectations: These are specific features and benefits customers want from our service. They can relate to behaviors (that is, being treated with respect and dignity, protecting confidentiality, and so on). They can relate to systems and processes (that is, the way we bill customers, the way we schedule them for tests, and the way we orient them to our services). They can also relate to the environment (that is, cleanliness, convenience of locations, ease of navigation). All of these preferences and wishes translate into expectations, which we need to understand and remember as we develop service standards.

Service Behaviors: These describe exactly what staff are supposed to do and say for and with customers. They describe in a common language what we mean by a service-oriented workforce. It's helpful to articulate these behaviors in the form of behavioral guidelines for all staff.

Job-Specific Service Behaviors: Most services and systems make explicit basic, generic service behaviors and communicate these as performance expectations of all staff. The truly service-oriented systems and services have gone the next step and fine-tuned these generic behaviors (applicable to all) and expanded on them with more specifics for people in each job. The result is that every employee in every job understands what he or she is supposed to do within that specific job to please customers. Tools that help turn generic service behaviors into job-specific service behaviors are protocols and scripts that spell out how the behaviors should be done (even with words to be used) in the staff members' specific roles.

Service Standards: These are promises your service makes to its customers. You set these standards based on knowledge of what your customers want most from your service, as well as from norms for service delivery in the marketplace. Standards change over time, since customer wants and market norms change also over time. These standards must, in some way, be measurable. For example, let's say you learn from patients that they want quick access to your service and that they want to be able to make appointments with their physician without having to wait a long time. Your service standard—based on your determination of what is doable and what your customers said they want—is "100 percent of our patients will be seen by a physician within 48 hours." Service standards are the measurable levels of performance you decide to achieve.

Service Targets: These are goals you establish because they are important to your customers and you have determined that reaching these goals will have a great impact on customer satisfaction. These are the service performance factors you want to improve on over time with specific levels you're aiming for. While your standard might be that people can get an appointment within 48 hours, your target might be more ambitious, such as, "Patients can get an appointment the same day!"

The Nine-Step Method

We'll walk you through the process of establishing high standards step-by-step with examples because it can be confusing. If it feels tedious, be patient, because there are big payoffs. Imagine your whole team clear about what they should be doing, and you with methods in hand for monitoring and measuring effectiveness.

The following nine-step process adds up to a comprehensive, powerful system of accountability for customer service. Each step, accompanied by tools, is explicated in the following sections.

Nine-Step Accountability Process

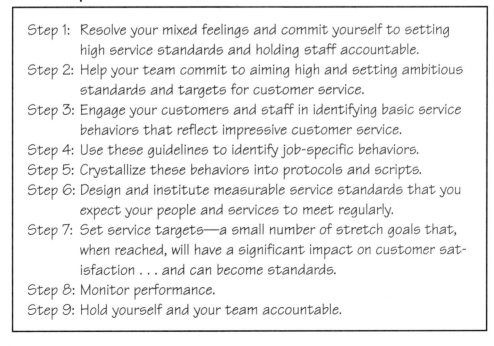

Step 1: Resolve your mixed feelings and commit yourself to setting high service standards and holding staff accountable.

Step 2: Help your team commit to aiming high and setting ambitious standards and targets for customer service.

Step 3: Engage your customers and staff in identifying basic service behaviors that reflect impressive customer service.

Step 4: Use these guidelines to identify job-specific behaviors.

Step 5: Crystallize these behaviors into protocols and scripts.

Step 6: Design and institute measurable service standards that you expect your people and services to meet regularly.

Step 7: Set service targets—a small number of stretch goals that, when reached, will have a significant impact on customer satisfaction . . . and can become standards.

Step 8: Monitor performance.

Step 9: Hold yourself and your team accountable.

Step 1: Resolve Mixed Feelings

The first step in the nine-step accountability process is to resolve your mixed feelings, commit yourself to setting high standards, and hold your staff accountable. Hopefully, you're an exception to the painful fact that the main impediment to raising standards lies within managers, not staff. Many, many managers have mixed feelings about raising standards. So, even when they do, they back away from enforcing them with the result that the standards fade into the sunset. How does this happen?

Consider this scenario: Manager Lee is frustrated with Herbie, a staff member who occasionally, when under a lot of pressure, mouths off to a customer. Usually, Herbie extends wonderful customer service to his customers. Lee wishes Herbie would control his occasional outbursts because they create havoc with customer satisfaction and problems for other staff. But Lee worries that maybe Herbie has too much pressure on him, or she wonders if maybe 100 percent consistent positive interactions with customers is too much to expect. More than once, Lee decides to confront Herbie about his behavior, but when the time comes, mixed feelings set in and Lee backs off, losing more sleep that night over her lack of courage.

When it comes to service behavior, Lee is not alone. Like many managers, she is plagued by ambivalence about whether she is justified in expecting better behavior from Herbie. The fact is, these mixed feelings stop Lee and other managers from raising the service standards to what they really need to be. Lee's standard is really this: I expect you to behave in an exemplary way to customers most of the time, except when you are feeling overly pressed. Who's perfect after all?

If you want to raise service standards, resolve your mixed feelings or you'll retreat when the time comes to insist on higher standards and enforce them. The tools presented in this section were designed to help you do just that.

Resolve Mixed Feelings

The purpose of this tool is to help you sort out the forces *interfering* with your ability to set and enforce higher standards.

Method

This tool is based on behavioral scientist Kurt Lewin's method called force-field analysis.

1. Copy the following chart as a worksheet for yourself.

Goal: Raising Standards

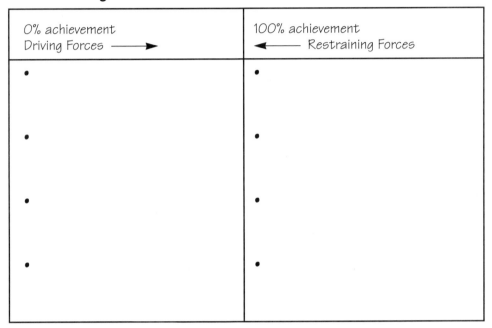

0% achievement Driving Forces ⟶	100% achievement ⟵ Restraining Forces
•	•
•	•
•	•
•	•

2. Complete the chart. In the left-hand column, list the forces driving or pushing you to set higher standards, both forces within yourself and outside yourself. In the right-hand column, list the forces restraining you or getting in the way of raising service standards, again including forces within you and outside of you.

3. Consider which driving forces you can increase and which will push you toward your goal of raising standards. Consider which restraining forces you can decrease, with the effect of eliminating obstacles to raising standards. Star one of each—one driving force that you can, through your own efforts, increase, and one restraining force that you can, through your own efforts, decrease. Here's an example. Let's say you enter under driving forces your recognition that there's a need to improve.

Goal: Raising Standards

0% achievement Driving Forces ———▶	100% achievement ◀——— Restraining Forces
• Commitment to customers • Commitment to staff development • Need for improvement	• I hate conflict! • I don't want to play police. • People don't share similar values and insights.

4. Make a plan to do it. Figure out how to follow through on one way to reduce a restraining force and one way to strengthen a driving force. The result will be that you will be closer to your goal of raising standards. Pursuing the example from above, if you identified a driving force as recognizing the need to improve, you could increase the strength of that driving force by getting information from others to confirm the need. Or closely watch that service so you can in no way escape seeing the pressing need to improve. And if you wrote under restraining forces that you're afraid raising standards will push you into the role of playing police, you might consider decreasing the strength of that restraining force by listing ways you can engage staff and customer feedback to help you hold people accountable. Then you're not alone in the police role. By increasing the driving force and decreasing the restraining force, you would push yourself toward your goal of getting mentally prepared to raise standards.

Remember that you can always adapt tools such as these to suit your situation. For example, talk to someone else who knows you well when completing the worksheet, because this person might see patterns in you that reveal restraining and driving forces. Also, engage this person's help in figuring out ways you can strengthen a driving force and reduce or weaken a restraining force. In our example, ask them, "What can I do to avoid having to play police once I set standards?"

Tips

- This tool can be helpful if you are a person who can change as a result of raising your awareness. Use it to think through the forces affecting what might be your paralysis about raising standards or your tendency to get tough with standards, but then back away when a particular employee falls short. Use this tool to sort out your motivations.

- Be sure to move on to the step of identifying one restraining force and one driving force to change, so that you can move yourself up the continuum toward feeling more comfortable about raising standards.

Talk Yourself Out of Your Own Way

This tool will help you replace self-talk that stops you from raising standards with self-talk that helps you raise them effectively. Use this tool if you get in your own way by saying to yourself things that have the effect of stopping you from intervening to raise standards.

Method

Copy the following worksheet and fill in the left-hand column. Then fill in the right-hand column. This chart includes an example.

Replace Unhelpful Self-Talk with Helpful Self-Talk

What do you say/think to yourself that stops you from intervening to raise service standards?	What could you say to yourself that would help you raise standards, not stop you from doing so?
• What right do I have to do this? • If I do this, I'll have to keep watch from now on! • I'm not perfect, so how can I expect my staff to be?	• I not only have the right to do this, I have the responsibility. • If I do this, I will have to keep watch, but over time, I will get the behavior our customers deserve. • It's true that no one's perfect, but I'm not expecting perfection. I'm asking for consistently better behavior to a standard that many people can easily meet.

Tip

- If you pinpoint a really helpful self-statement, write it on a card and put it on your desk for a few weeks. Read it daily and try to imprint it on your brain, so you'll think it when you need to. A friend can help you generate constructive alternatives after you've identified your current self-talk.

Step 2: Help Your Staff Commit

The second step in the accountability process is to help your team commit to aiming high and setting ambitious standards for customer service. OK, so you are committed! But what about your staff? If you can't enthuse them about the whole idea of raising the standards to impress their customers, you're going to be tugging and prodding, pushing and pulling. The following tools help you touch the chords of motivation—the personal missions and aspirations of your staff—so that they join you in raising the standards.

Who Benefits?

This tool helps staff become more aware of the importance of raising standards and how this can benefit them.[1]

Method

1. Divide the group into small teams of three to five people.
2. Ask the teams to generate numerous ways that different stakeholder groups can benefit from the deliverance of top-notch, impressive service. Have people consider such groups as the following:
   —You
   —Our team
   —Patients
   —Payers
   —The organization
   —The community
3. Give the teams about 10 minutes to generate their lists and ask them to share with the larger group. Capture the information on a flipchart.

4. Ask, "Of the benefits listed, which do you feel strongest about and why?"

Tips

- The purpose of this exercise is to get the group talking about what they have personally to gain. We usually talk about the survival of the team, the system, or the community. We also spend time thinking about what the customer stands to gain, but we don't spend as much time discussing what staff have to gain. And if we do talk about the payoffs and benefits, the discussions seem to be pretty superficial. "Which do you feel strongest about and why?" That's the most important question. It provides an opportunity to go deeper, to encourage people to picture how it would feel to work with a team known for service greatness. Encourage discussion of such issues as pride, self-esteem, personal growth, and development in addition to the more obvious ones like enhanced teamwork and less stress.

Feel free to participate yourself. In fact, if you get personal, staff are more likely to do so, too.

Think of a Place

This tool helps staff think about what truly great service looks like. It will help to create a common vision within the group and reinforce the fact that, as consumers, we know what great service looks like.

Method

1. Tell the group, "You're going to spend a few minutes discussing great service, beginning with what it looks like."
2. Ask people to spend a few minutes thinking about one place they've been that has impressed them with its service. This place could be anywhere—their hairdresser, the dry cleaner, a store, a restaurant, a hotel, or another medical facility.
3. Ask staff to get together with a partner and jot down some of the things that impressed them about the service using the handout What Wows You?

Handout: What Wows You?

Think of a place you like a lot because of the great service they provide to customers. List the things that you like the most about that place:

-

-

-

-

Why are these things important to you?

How many and which of these things involve systems and processes?

How many and which of these things have to do with the physical environment?

How many and which of these things have to do with the people and the way they treat you as a customer?

What, specifically, do staff there do that wows or impresses you?

4. Ask partners to share their ideas with the rest of the group, while you capture the common themes on flipchart paper.
5. Have the group look over the list and identify the systems and processes that support excellent service as well as the behaviors—the things people say and do to satisfy customers.
6. Process the activity by discussing the following questions:
   —Which items were most important to you as a customer?
   —How is staff able to make these happen?
   —Are these similar to what our customers want from us?
   —Which ones are easy and hard for us to deliver?

Tips

- The important thing is to have staff think about the importance of great service to them as a consumer. They obviously make choices about where to spend their time and their money based on the service they receive, and their customers are no different.
- As you hear staff discuss very basic things people do to wow customers, reinforce that these are the same regardless of the service or industry.
- If no one else makes the critical point, make it yourself. The difference between the places that people think of as superior and other places is that the former provide specific service features better and more consistently than their competitors.

Moving from *Good* to *Great*

This tool has two purposes:

1. To help staff identify the very real and important difference between GOOD and GREAT.
2. To help staff think of the specific things they can do to really impress customers.

Method

1. Ask staff to brainstorm a list of typical customer interactions that occur daily.

2. Ask small groups to choose one example from the list and prepare two very short skits. The skits should present the everyday
interaction in two different ways. The first should demonstrate
good or acceptable behavior on the part of staff. The second
should demonstrate the same interaction, but this time the staff
member should do as many things as possible to really impress
the customer.

3. After each pair of skits, the rest of the group shares their reactions to the following questions:
   —What did the staff member do in the second interaction to
   make a big difference?
   —What difference do you think this made to the customer?
   What else could the staff member have done to really impress
   the customer?

4. At the end of all the skits, ask the group for general themes and
reactions.

Tips

- If you think that your team will have difficulty coming up with
good examples of everyday interactions with customers, think of
a few ahead of time, write them on slips of paper, put them in a
hat, and let small groups each pick one out of the hat.

- Make sure you make the main point very explicitly and clearly.
The little things we do make a big difference. These little things
need to become the standard rather than the exception. Good
really isn't good enough.

This is not supposed to be a training session on dealing with difficult people or difficult situations, but rather an awareness raiser
on how much better we can be in our everyday moments of truth
with customers. For this reason, make sure the skits are about simple interactions—skits, not three-act plays.

Step 3: Identify Impressive Customer Service Behaviors

For step 3 engage your customers and staff in identifying basic service behaviors reflective of impressive customer service. To do this,
establish basic behavioral guidelines for customer service based on

what customers want and staff can deliver. Without these, staff members operate from their own assumptions about what they should be doing . . . different assumptions that lead to different levels of performance. With that, how can you possibly expect consistent performance at a high level?

To begin, you know that standards for customer service need to be driven by customer expectations. To find out what customers expect, consult them. But you can't do this yourself. You don't have time! So involve staff. They need to find out what will impress their customers. With this information, they will have a better grip on what their customers want and will feel much more committed to meeting their expectations than they would if you, as intermediary, spoke for customers. Use this next tool to involve your staff in finding out their customers' service priorities.

What Do Customers Expect?

This tool helps you to do the following:

- Find out from customers what matters most to them about your service.
- Use customer input to help the team determine what they should be doing and how they should be doing it in order to impress customers.
- Have staff facilitate and own the process.

Method

1. Invite staff to join you in asking customers for information about what satisfies and impresses them the most when needing help or service from your team.
2. Set up a two-week period during which staff gather information from customers.
3. Give each staff member an assigned customer group (or one they volunteer to contact), making sure all customer groups (that is, patients/families, payers, referral sources, internal customers, or other customers) are going to be contacted by some staff.
4. Give each staff member ten copies of this customer contact form and ask them to use it as a guide to recording their answers when gathering information from customers.

Customer Contact Form

Introduction: We are asking our customers for information about what they want most when they come to our clinic/service/department/organization, so we can take steps to better satisfy our customers. I have three questions to ask you. Can you please spare three minutes to answer my questions?

1. When you come in or call our [clinic, HMO, office, service, department], what can we do to satisfy you with our service?

   Examples of answers staff might receive:
   - People answer the phone promptly and don't put me on hold for a long time.
   - I can get an appointment right away.
   - I would see my provider within 15 minutes of my scheduled appointment.

2. How would we do that? What would we be doing to meet these expectations? How would staff be acting or behaving?

   Examples:
   - Someone would tell me how long I have to wait, if there's a wait; they wouldn't wait for me to hound them.
   - I would be welcomed with a smile and warmth from everyone I meet.

3. What would we need to do to impress you—not just satisfy you, but impress you?

   Examples:
   - If I consistently got seen at the time of my appointment.
   - If the nurse and doctor didn't rush me but took the time to answer my questions.

5. Have each staff member make ten contacts, being sure to contact all of your customer groups, so that you all develop a clear picture of how to impress all the customers your team serves.
6. Bring staff together to share their findings and develop together a summary list of service behaviors their customers want and expect. Keep these on hand for when staff proceed to crystallize behavior guidelines for the team.

Tips

- Help staff prepare! Provide them with practice times so they can rehearse with each other.
- Be sure to have staff members contact representatives of all customer groups, so you'll have input into what impresses each group.
- Make it clear to staff how to select the customers they contact and give them a chance to practice their initial pitch if they are hesitant to make their contacts.
- Also, arrange for times when staff can compare notes about the process and learn tips from each other about how to be effective (good questioners and grateful, skillful listeners) in their data gathering from customers.
- While this activity takes time and work up front, it proves to be a very positive experience for staff. They end up feeling connected to their customers, they feel informed, and their customers have faces and voices that influence staff behavior and attitudes. Also, many staff members find the role of interviewer a job-enhancing diversion from their regular service responsibilities.

Engage All Staff in Setting Basic Behavioral Guidelines

Equipped with customer expectations in hand, the next step is to develop basic service behaviors—guidelines that spell out the generic behaviors (those applicable to everybody) that impress customers. Why bother? Because these behaviors aren't clear to everyone. Without a shared understanding of appropriate behavior, the normal curve takes over. Some staff are awful in their behavior. Some are wonderful. And many, many are in the middle of the range. By spelling out key behaviors expected of everyone, you'll still see a normal curve of behavior, but that normal curve occurs around a much higher standard. More people know what's expected of them and more people do it, still with some variation around the edges.

Method

Here's how your ultimate product of service behaviors might look. This one applies to an ambulatory care service.

Service Behaviors (House Rules): Community Care Center

1. Welcome warmly. First impressions last. Make eye contact, smile, and extend a warm welcome. Introduce yourself. Call people by name.
2. Put people at ease. Reach out with friendly words and gestures. Extend a few words of concern. Convey confidence. This is what people remember.
3. Keep people informed. Tell people what to expect. Invite questions. Check back and apologize for delays. People will be calmer and grateful.
4. Anticipate. You'll often know what people need before they have to ask. Don't wait. Act first.
5. Respond quickly. When people are worried and waiting, every minute is an hour.
6. Respect privacy and confidentiality. Watch what you say and where you say it. Respect and protect a person's rights.
7. Respect patients' dignity. That person could be your child, your relative, or your friend. Give choices. Cover people up. Knock as you enter. Respect the PERSON.
8. Take initiative. Just because it's not your job doesn't mean you can't help or find someone who can.
9. Treat patients as adults. Your words and tone should not insult.
10. Keep it quiet. Noise disturbs when people are anxious. Remember where you are. Show consideration. Remind each other. Keep it professional.
11. Listen. When people complain, don't be defensive. Hear them out and show understanding. Give alternatives. Do all you can to make things right.
12. Follow through. Own the problem. Tie up loose ends. Close the loop with the customer.
13. Help each other and you help a patient.
14. Take care on the phone. Our reputation's on the line. Sound pleasant, listen with understanding, and help.
15. Maintain a professional image. You're part of a long, proud health care tradition. Look the part.

What Will It Take?

This tool helps your staff to do the following:[2]

- Translate customer expectations into specific behaviors
- Identify opportunities for growth and improvement
- Make sure that behavioral expectations mean the same to everyone on the team
- Develop shared ownership of higher expectations

Method

1. Review with your team what everyone learned when they talked with customers about the service behaviors that customers care about when using their service—features like keeping the noise down, getting respect, being listened to, and the like. Place one on each of several flipchart pages around the room.
2. Ask the group to create a sentence or two under each that clarifies and expands on what that service behavior implies.
3. Break the large group into smaller groups with one group standing in front of each flipchart.
4. Give the small groups 10 minutes to flesh out specifics related to the behavior on their flipchart, including examples and how-to's that reflect the work they do in their roles with customers.
5. After 10 minutes, have the groups rotate to another flipchart. Ask them to look over the list done by the previous group and find ways to make it more specific and more complete. They should refine the list as they see it.
6. After another ten minutes, have groups rotate again to another flipchart. This time, the small groups should look at the list in front of them and think about editing it so that they push for excellence, dazzle customers, and stretch for the best they can be.
7. Groups rotate one more time and give another list a final once-over with an eye to fine-tuning language, collapsing redundant information, and adding final touches. The result should be a very complete list under each heading—a list that spells out what employees could be doing to demonstrate that behavior.
8. These groups then look over their list and prepare to give a five-minute presentation of it to the large group. Their goals are to explain why this behavior is important now and in the future,

what employees need to do to demonstrate it fully and consistently, ways individuals are currently doing and not doing this with customers, and finally recommendations for improvement.

9. Now you need to fine-tune the service behaviors with the goal of creating a polished list. Consider developing a representative subcommittee to do the work—what we call a service behaviors team. Give your whole staff a chance to make final recommendations and changes, so you end up with an endorsement by all staff of the basic service behaviors that apply to everyone.

Tips

- If your group is small, have groups as small as two people. Otherwise groups of three or four are advisable. If you don't have enough groups to assign one behavior to each, give each group several behaviors to address.
- Because this method engages everyone in looking at the behaviors and thinking them through, it has a powerful awareness-raising effect that helps you raise the bar in addition to articulating clear behavioral guidelines. Take the time to do this.

What's Next?

This last exercise is a great way to help staff see the opportunities they have to impress their customers, but most groups will only be able to come up with what you're likely to consider a rough draft. Now you need to fine-tune the service behaviors with the goal of creating a polished list of those behaviors that you want staff to focus on and that truly reflect your expectations.

Work with a Service Behaviors Team to Fine-Tune Service Guidelines

This can be done in one or two marathon work sessions or in a series of meetings. The advantage of marathon work sessions is that once people get involved and warmed up, they are more efficient and productive than they are in a series of short meetings, each of which requires warming up once again to the task.

Method

1. Before the meeting starts, take the lists of service behaviors brainstormed previously by both customers and staff, and write each one on a Post-It note. Stick these to the wall in the meeting room (or if they don't stick, spread them out on a huge table).

2. Welcome the team members and explain that you are asking them to represent their internal and external customers in the process.

3. Ask the team to look at the potpourri of service behaviors on the Post-It notes, reminding them that these reflect the input of customers and staff. The task now is to categorize them using a technique called affinity charting. Ask the team to stand up and, using one wall of the room, move the Post-Its around to form clusters of related behaviors; then they should together name each cluster. You'll probably end up with several categories with a mishmash of descriptive words, behaviors, and so on under each. The task then is to tighten up each category: crystallize the category name, remove redundancy and items that do nothing more than paraphrase the category name, and keep under the category every behavior that falls within it. You might end up with several categories and behaviors under each. Each will look something like this:

Communicates Effectively

- Tells me if I have to wait
- Makes eye contact
- Smiles

Uses Professional Phone Tactics

- Answers with their name
- Doesn't just put me on hold without asking
- Transfers me to the right person

---

4. Ask the group whether there are any categories missing—any aspects of service that have been omitted, and if so, add them. Then do a quick brainstorming of behaviors under each.

5. Figure out with the team how to go the next steps—to examine the category name, making it very clear, and to develop the list of top-priority behaviors associated with each category. Do people want to work together in additional meetings or divide up the categories, assigning one or more to each of several pairs? Or does the group want to brainstorm on each category, asking what behaviors are missing, and then prioritize the big five behaviors for each category? Give all of it to someone on the team who's known as the writer or wordsmith for final polish.

Variations

- If you have an old set of perfectly good behavioral guidelines or service behaviors, have staff look at them after they have brainstormed based on customer expectations. Don't just adapt them, because they might be either outdated or have been developed based on staff input, not customer input.
- If your service or organization has a set of values that are meant to drive development of service behaviors, use your values as the service categories and build behaviors related to them as shown in the example below. Note, however, that your current values might not have been developed based on customers' main expectations.

Value	Behavior Guideline	Behaviors
Responsiveness to customers	Listens	• Invites customers to talk • Listens patiently • Checks their understanding • Listens openly without being defensive

Tips

- This task starts slowly and then speeds up as people get the knack. You'll find that they'll be encouraged by their own progress.
- Provide a thesaurus and dictionary to the team, so they can have access to alternative words. Or show them how to access these resources on a computer.

We're on Board!

This tool will assist you in developing shared ownership of the service behaviors by inviting staff input before the service behaviors team casts the behaviors list in stone.

Method

1. Reconvene the service behaviors team after people have produced a draft of the service behaviors and invite nit-picking!
   —Improve the wording of each behavior, so it's clear, clear, clear.
   —Add missing behaviors.
   —Refine the wording of the behaviors.
   —Remove behaviors that people don't see as top priority.
2. End up with a manageable number of behaviors, clearly stated.
3. Type a draft.
4. Present the draft to staff in a meeting or circulate the draft with a memo and instructions to buddy with a coworker to review it and make further suggestions.
5. If you use a memo, invite people to respond in writing or by contacting any member of the service behaviors team with their feedback and suggestions. Ask them the following:
   —What's not clear?
   —What's missing?
   —What shouldn't be there?
   —What suggestions do you have?
   —How can we improve the wording?
   Better yet, have the service behaviors team present the draft to all staff in a meeting or hold small get-togethers with subgroups to review the draft before the meeting with all staff:
   —Have each team member participate in the presentation by taking one or two behavior categories and explaining the thinking and process behind each.
   —Explain the process the team went through to draft the behaviors.
   —Ask for feedback from all staff after each category is presented and take flipchart notes.
6. Have the service behaviors team refine the basic service behaviors based on the feedback and create a final document.
7. Type into a snazzy format.

Tips

- Feature members of the service behaviors team at every step. This way, others on your team will see that their colleagues are involved. Some might be all the more likely to contribute and help a colleague too.
- The key in developing behaviors is to get very, very specific. If you stay general, you don't actually influence behavior change. If people can't picture the behavior when they read the wording, encourage people to go back to the drawing board to get more specific.
- Involve frontline staff from the start. They will have to instigate these behaviors in interactions with customers, and they're likely to resent behavior guidelines handed to them from on high.

It's an achievement to crystallize the service behaviors list, but the process doesn't end there. Many services in the past have gone this far and been disappointed by their outcomes. They didn't help staff apply the behaviors to people's jobs. They didn't get job specific. That's the essential next step.

Step 4: Use These Guidelines to Identify Job-Specific Behaviors

So far, you found out from customers what they want and need. If your system or service didn't have a generic list of service behaviors, you pulled these together. You used various tools to flesh these out, making them clearer, less redundant, and more specific. And you helped staff approve and own these behaviors, so that everyone is on the same wavelength.

Now help staff figure out what these service behaviors mean to them, in their jobs, in the work that each person does, and with their specific customers. Some staff just don't figure this out on their own. They might be trapped in or blinded by their routines and fail to see opportunities to demonstrate these key behaviors. Other staff members resist changing their behavior because they just don't want to. When pressed to change or when confronted, they use the excuse, "I wasn't clear on what I was supposed to do in my job." If you don't take the next step of helping them see how the service behaviors apply to their jobs, they are justified in doing so (as much as this might irritate you!).

Apply the Behaviors to My Job

This tool will focus staff on their service behaviors and help them to clarify their application to specific roles.

Method

Meet with staff by job category or with all staff in a staff meeting. If your service is large and you have people in supervisory jobs, these supervisors can hold the meetings.

1. Give each person a copy of their job description and a copy of the service behaviors.
2. Divide them into pairs and have pairs interview each other about how these service behaviors apply to their specific jobs. Ask them to match up their job descriptions with the behaviors, finding opportunities in their daily work to exhibit these behaviors.

Interview Questions: What Do These Behaviors Mean to You?

- Which of these behaviors do you like doing?
- Which do you find easy to do?
- Which do you find hard to do?
- Which don't you believe in doing at all?
- In your job, where do you see the opportunities for engaging in these behaviors with the effect of impressing customers?
- On which of these behaviors do you think you have room for improvement? Which would enhance your performance and effectiveness?

3. Invite their questions with an eye to making it clear how the behaviors apply within their individual jobs.

Tips

- If you have more than one person in each position, have these people work together.
- Also, create opportunities for people in different jobs to review the work of the job-specific groups to make additional suggestions.

Step 5: Crystallize These Behaviors into Job-Specific Protocols and Scripts

If you want to achieve dramatic breakthroughs in service behavior, go the next step and, using the service behaviors as guidelines, engage staff in working out service protocols and scripts that build these behaviors into predictable, reliable everyday routines.

Service behaviors provide a backdrop for doing the more meticulous work of developing service protocols and scripts for specific jobs. Service protocols are step-by-step, sequential guidelines for behavior in specific situations. They tell you exactly how you're supposed to do the task or job. For example, consider this job-specific protocol for greeting people:

Sample Protocol: Department of Physical Therapy Secretary Protocol

---

Greeting Initial Outpatients/Electromyography (EMG) Patients at the Window

1. Look up, establish eye contact, smile, and say, "Good morning/afternoon, may I help you?" Use a friendly tone of voice.
2. If it's an outpatient, say, "May I have your name please?"
3. Respond, "Oh, yes, Ms./Mr./Mrs. _____. I'm glad to see you here for therapy/an EMG. Please come in and have a seat to the left, and I'll be right with you. I have some forms you will need to fill out, and I need to make a copy of your insurance card."
4. Speak to the patient quietly and directly to obtain the necessary information and fill out forms. Take them into the office or a private area if you need to discuss insurance and other patients are in the waiting room. Ask if they would like help filling out forms. (If so, help! Offer to do the writing.)
5. Say, "I'll be back in a few moments to see whether you have any questions." (And check back with them shortly.)
6. After the person fills out the forms, if the therapist is not yet ready for the patient, tell the patient how long it will be. For instance, "Your therapist is working with another patient and isn't quite ready. I hope you don't mind waiting about _____ minutes?"
7. When the patient can go back to therapy, go out to the waiting area and address the patient by name. Say, "Mr./Ms./Mrs. _____? [Name of therapist] is ready for you now. Let me show you the way to his/her area."

8. While you're walking, focus on the patient and connect to him or her with small talk or say, "You'll be in good hands with [name of therapist]."

9. Whenever possible, walk the patient back to the outpatient area or request an aide.

10. For an EMG patient, say, "The doctor will be with you in about _____ minutes. In the meantime, I'll be in the office if you need anything at all."

11. If the wait will be long, apologize for the delay and see if there is anything you can get the patient. Update the patient about the wait at least every five minutes.

12. When you reach the therapist, introduce the patient to the therapist: "Mrs./Mr./Ms., I'd like you to meet _____, who will be your therapist today," and wish the patient a good day.

Reprinted, with permission, from the Albert Einstein Healthcare Network © 1996

Scripts include the exact words people are supposed to use. For instance, staff might have a script for explaining a certain charge to a patient, or a script of a greeting they're supposed to use when they see a doctor approaching. Service protocols and scripts specify in precise terms the behaviors and words expected of staff. By developing protocols and scripts with an eye to aiming for excellence—to impress customers, not just satisfy them—you can reach an awe-inspiring level of service.

Some staff resist protocols and scripts. They'll accuse you of wanting them to become automatons. They'll accuse you of failing to respect individual differences and individual styles. They'll express their concern that if they follow scripts, they'll sound phony. They're right to express these concerns, but these concerns should not stop you in your tracks. There are answers.

Scripts and protocols don't create automatons. They create consistency at a high standard. If you don't reach this level of specificity, you will see too much variation in service delivery, wide variation around an implicit, not explicit, standard. Protocols and scripts still allow for individual differences in style within a range. It's true that they rule out differences that engender different, sometimes inferior, levels of customer satisfaction. Protocols and scripts say, "At least do this much, and if you can do even more to satisfy your customers, feel free to use your creativity, ingenuity, and individual pizzazz to go the extra mile. But at least do this much, and your customers will be impressed."

To staff who think protocols and scripts make staff sound phony, tell them that sounding genuine when following the protocol or script is in itself part of the protocol or script. A phony voice or robotic style reflects failure to implement the protocol!

As luck would have it, you'll find many staff relieved to have the clarity about what's expected of them that only protocols and scripts provide.

Persist in developing service protocols and scripts because the payoffs are astounding. Just visit the Ritz Carlton and hear every person introduce themselves to you and call you by name often. And call the Ritz Carlton and feel the good feeling of hearing everyone respond, with enthusiasm and warmth, "My pleasure" when you thank anyone for transferring your call or giving you information. It's service protocols and scripts that have made Ritz Carlton service consistently outstanding in every facility in the world, and it's protocols and scripts that have won the Ritz Carlton every national and international award for outstanding service.

Here is a sequential process for developing job-specific service protocols and scripts. Staff involvement is critical at every action step.

Action 1: Identify the critical steps along the customer's pathway through your service.

Action 2: Interview customers about what they want from staff at each step and what staff would need to do at each step in order to impress them.

Action 3: For each staff responsibility in the right-hand column, identify the actions and behaviors (and for scripts, the exact words) that will be sure to impress customers.

Action 4: Codify these behaviors and words into service protocols and scripts and develop job aids to remind staff of how they're supposed to perform each task.

Action 5: Sort the protocols and scripts by position and give those that relate to each specific position to the people in that position. Label them Job-Specific Service Protocols/Scripts.

Action 6: Build staff skills in following these protocols and scripts by providing training, practice, and feedback.

This systematic approach results in wonderful protocols and scripts for staff, with the added payoff of providing you with instructions you can give to new employees to equip them to do their new jobs. The message is "This is how we do things here."

Action 1: Identify the Critical Steps along the Customer's Pathway through Your Service

First, organize staff teams or pairs to map the patient's pathway through your service and define staff responsibilities at each step. Then on paper, make a chart with two columns. Label the column on the left Steps along Patient Pathway. In the right-hand column, write Main Staff Responsibilities. For instance, in a mammography service, this map might look like this:

Steps along Patient Pathway	Main Staff Responsibilities
Approaches front desk to check in	• Welcomes patient • Tells patient what's next
Goes to registration person	• Hands off patient to registration person
Sits in waiting area	• Explains wait
Gets taken to changing area	• Tells patient staff is ready and directs to changing area • Shows where to undress • Explains extent of undressing • Explains what to do when finished
Disrobes and waits for directions	• Watches to see when patient is ready and tells patient what's next (whether to wait or go to procedure room)
Goes to procedure room and meets technologist	• Introduces patient to technologist • Technologist welcomes, warms up patient • Explains procedure
Has mammogram	• Walks patient through procedure • Explains • Invites/addresses questions • Makes small talk to ease anxiety

Goes back to waiting area while pictures are checked	• Leads patient back to waiting area • Explains need to wait for picture check before dressing • Explains time involved
Learns whether retake is needed or if she can dress	• Explains if pictures are OK or not • Tells woman whether she can dress or come back to procedure room for retake
If she can dress, learns how she'll hear results and that she can leave when ready	• Explains what happens next • Explains how and when woman will learn of results • Clarifies whether woman can leave after getting dressed
Learns of results	• Passes pictures to radiologist for review • Documents as needed • Notifies referring doctor(s) of results • Follows procedures for notifying woman

Now you have a fairly good idea of what your staff's responsibilities are, and you can move to the next step.

Action 2: Interview Customers

Interview customers about what they want from staff at each step and what staff would need to do at each step in order to impress them.

Method

1. Engage members of your team in finding out from customers what would impress them at each step through their experience with your service.
2. With the pathway in hand, interview a few former or current patients or conduct focus groups with customers to find out what they wish staff would do and how they wish staff would behave at each step.

Interview and Focus Group Instructions

1. Introduce yourself and your purpose: "We're trying to improve our services, so that people who choose us for service get the top-notch service they deserve. We're asking your help. I want to find out from you what you *wish* your experience here would be like. I can promise that we will use what we learn to improve our services for you and our other customers."

2. Check the pathway: "Let me show you the steps most patients go through when they come here for the service you came for. (Show the steps). Does this reflect the steps you went through, or are these steps different from the ones you went through when you came here for service?" (Add any steps they suggest; alter the flowchart according to their modifications.)

3. Find out what would impress the customer at each step in the pathway. Go through the steps in the pathway one by one and also name the staff's responsibilities at each step: "Now, let me find out your thoughts. I want to know two things:
   —"What bothered you even slightly at each step?
   —"What could our staff have done differently or better?" (Probe for details by asking such questions as, "What exactly did you want to know that staff didn't explain? How could we have made that handoff smoother?")

4. Thank people profusely for their help and reinforce that you will use the results to improve service for customers in the future.

Here's what customer input might sound like:

Step along Patient Pathway: Patient Gets Taken to Changing Area

Main Staff Responsibilities	Patient Response
Tells patient staff is ready and directs to changing area	"I wish the person who did this didn't call my name across the room. I wish they'd come over to me, look me in the eye, say my name, and tell me who's going to see me next and when . . . and what I need to do about changing clothes."

Shows where to undress	"I wish there was a lock on the door, so I wouldn't be afraid of someone barging in."
Explains extent of undress needed	"I never know whether I have to take everything off, or just what's on top, and can I keep on my jewelry?"
Explains what to do when finished	"You're kind of left in the dark about what to do when you're in a robe. Are you supposed to go find a technologist or sit there or stay in the room with the door open or what? I just hang around feeling unsure."

This input makes it quite clear what staff need to do and say (and how to say it) to improve this step of the service process. Imagine if the staff member could anticipate every anxiety and question the woman might have and preempt it by saying all the right things? All the right things—that's the service protocol that needs to get developed in the next step.

 Tips

- Take copious notes about what the customers say for each step in the pathway. These notes help you to remember what the customer wants when you craft the details you need to build great service protocols.
- Consult customers to get this information by having each staff member interview a couple of former patients or by inviting a group of former patients to lunch or dinner and using a group discussion format.
- You probably have someone in your organization who can serve as facilitator. The key to both interviewing and running focus groups effectively is that the facilitator asks questions and listens and does not react or respond to any of the answers—just listen, listen, listen and probe, probe, probe, and finally thank, thank, thank people for helping to make your service better.

Action 3: Identify Actions and Behaviors

For each staff responsibility, identify the actions and behaviors (and if you're scripting, the exact words) that will be sure to impress customers. It is vital to engage staff in developing protocols and scripts for every step in their customers' pathway through the service.

Method

1. Divide up the steps in the customer's experience and assign a few steps to each of several staff teams or pairs.
2. Give them the job of using the input from customers to identify protocols and scripts for doing each responsibility in an impressive way. For each step along the customer's pathway through the service, staff need to answer these questions:
   —What should we do? In what order?
   —What should we say?
   —What shouldn't we do or say?
3. Show examples, so staff understand the task and the degree of specificity needed. For instance, in the mammography example, for the step in the patient's pathway called "Gets taken to changing area," the design team would examine the customer input and build protocols or step-by-step instructions for the staff person who routinely fulfills that responsibility.

 Tips

- Make sure every team working on protocols has a member who can go beyond platitudes to pinpoint behavior. Or, arrange for a roving coach.
- Some managers arrange for a protocol design work session during which all teams work simultaneously in the same room on their protocols, making it possible to ask each other for advice and suggestions along the way.

Action 4: Codify These Behaviors into Service Protocols

Now is the time for editing and formatting so that every staff member has a user-friendly crib sheet that spells out behavior for their steps in the service process. Use scripts and job aids to remind staff of what they're supposed to do and say during each step in the customer's pathway through the service.

Method

Craft a job aid using the information you've gathered in the previous action steps. Here's an example of a job aid that shows the service protocol for one very important, very anxiety-producing step in the mammography service cycle:

Mammography Clerks' Protocol for Walking a Woman from the Reception Area to the Changing Room

1. Welcome the patient warmly. Walk up to the patient in waiting area. (Don't call out to her.) Call her by name, and introduce yourself and say why you're there. For example, "Hello, are you Mrs. Corbin? Mrs. Corbin, I'm Maxine, and I'm here to show you the way to the cubby where you can change into a robe."

2. Show her the way and connect to her as a person along the way. Walk close to her; don't dart ahead. While you're walking, tell her the name of the technologist who will do the procedure and express your confidence in the technologist. For example, "When you're ready, Helen Locke, the technologist, will do your mammogram. You'll be in good hands with Helen!" Make other small talk along the way if needed—about the weather, the news.

3. In the changing area, show the woman to a specific room, saying, "Here's an available room."

4. Explain undressing. "You'll need to take off everything on the top, including your jewelry and underwear. You can leave on your slacks and shoes."

5. Tell her how she can have privacy. "While you're in there, you can lock the door from the inside if you'd like."

6. Tell her what to do when finished. "Then, when you're ready, please come out and have a seat in one of these chairs over here and your technologist, Helen, will come for you."

7. Tell her what she needs to do to protect her possessions, so she won't feel anxious about possible theft. "Also, I suggest that you bring your purse with you, but everything else you can leave in here with the door closed. They'll be perfectly safe here."

8. Invite questions. "Do you have any questions at this point?" Say a gracious good-bye. If you won't see the woman again, say, "I might not see you on your way out, so I'll say good-bye now. It was very nice meeting you."

Tips

- If you have good writers on hand, ask them to help in the editing process to tighten the protocols.
- Build in a feedback step during which teams circulate drafts of their protocols to each other and also show them to or try them out on customers and invite feedback and suggestions.

Action 5: Create Job-Specific Service Protocols

Now you have protocols and scripts galore. In this step, sort them so that each staff member has just the ones he or she needs. Sort the protocols by position and give those that relate to each specific position to the people in that position. Label them Job-Specific Service Protocols.

Method

1. Have a small group perform this step. Ask them to sort all of the protocols to be followed by people in each position into a protocol booklet, preferably loose-leaf for easy access, upgrading, and rearrangement. You'll end up with many protocols per position.
2. Have staff in each position sequence these in a way that makes sense for them, chronologically or by customer group.

Tips

- Make sure staff in each position have a chance to further refine the protocols that apply to them.
- The reason for using a loose-leaf notebook is that protocols should not be seen as cast in stone. The more staff are encouraged to fine-tune them as they use them, the more ownership people will feel in their own protocols and in their resulting excellent performance.
- Invite staff to design a cover for the protocol notebooks, a cover that, when seen by customers, makes a positive impression.

You're not finished yet. Staff need support in using the protocols effectively.

Action 6: Provide Training, Practice, and Feedback

Build staff skills in following these protocols by providing training, practice, and feedback. At first, staff are likely to find their protocols and scripts awkward. They'll feel stilted and mechanical. With protocols in hand, staff need to try them out and become comfortable with them until they feel routine. In this step, help staff internalize the protocols and scripts so that they can use them with comfort and effectiveness.

Method

1. Create a comfortable practice setting. Ask people to pair up and try out their protocols on each other. Encourage people to invite feedback and use the feedback not only to improve their own effectiveness in following the protocols, but also to make further refinements in the protocols themselves.
2. Develop a buddy system for mutual observation and coaching on the job.
3. Also, establish a habit-building period—at least three weeks long—for an on-the-job trial run of the protocols. After that, reconvene staff to formally assess the protocols and make needed revisions.

Tips

- Build support for staff to try out their protocols and actually use them repetitively on the job. If they don't use them, and use them, and use them again, they will not internalize the new habits in line with the newly raised standards.
- Some staff will complain that the protocols cause them to lose spontaneity. Emphasize that they don't have to use the exact words in the protocols. They just have to find words for fulfilling each function specified by customers as important. Scripts provide examples of effective words in case people don't want to come up with their own or for use when they're having a bad day. Instead of trusting themselves to use positive words, they may at times want to fall back on words sure to be effective.
- These protocols are fantastic orientation devices for new staff. When you have new employees, give them the protocols and say, "This is how we do things here!"

- How to sustain use of the protocols? That's a matter of constant reminders through observations and coaching, and also use of basic accountability principles.

Step 6: Design and Institute Measurable Service Standards

So far, we talked about behaviors and protocols that individuals are expected to follow in order to satisfy or impress customers. But behaviors and protocols are not one and the same as standards. Standards are different. They apply to the team. Standards establish the level of service the team commits itself to provide in order to satisfy or impress their customers. These standards must be quantitative (such as, "Keep people waiting no longer than 10 minutes" or "Introduce ourselves to 100 percent of our new customers").

Sometimes service standards relate to specific staff behaviors (like introducing yourself to 100 percent of your new customers), and sometimes they relate to your service product (such as, "Support people's care once they go home by calling 100 percent of discharged patients within 48 hours of their return home").

Set standards with staff, so that you can be sure to satisfy your customers' main expectations. The competitive edge lies in satisfying customer needs better than your competitors can and making sure your customers know it. By setting and enforcing standards or defining the sure things that customers will get when they opt for your services, your staff have clear requirements to fulfill and your customers know and believe the promises or commitments you're willing to make for their sakes.

Customers' Priorities Sensor

This tool helps to prioritize customers' stated expectations to establish service standards.

Earlier in this chapter, you found a tool that helped you consult customers to find out their main expectations of your service. Now, revisit the results and set standards related to their expectations.

Method

1. Lay out customer expectations on a chart.
2. Engage staff in discussing what it would take to meet each expectation.
3. Work on reaching agreement on what achievable level of service would meet customer expectations at the very least or better yet impress customers. End up with a chart that looks something like this chart from Saint Mary's Hospital in Green Bay, Wisconsin.

Saint Mary's Service Standards

Patient Expectations	Service Standards
ENT/Orthopedics • Prepare you for your care at home • Provide a 24-hour prescription dose • Provide competent staff • Communicate with patient/family • Offer continuity of care	• 100% of patients will receive teaching booklets • 100% of patients will be offered flat pack • Lidocaine wheel will be used for IV starts 90% of the time • Patient/family will be informed of reason for delays. • 100% of caregivers will introduce themselves
Gastrointestinal Unit • Have good physician interaction • Keep you informed during your stay • Prepare you for care at home	• Written results to referring physician within 24 hours. • 100% of patients will be discharged with written results. • Patients will be contacted every 15 minutes • 100% of patients will receive follow-up call, including weekends within _____ time frame
First Care • Keep you informed during your stay. • Provide a 24-hour prescription dose. • Be efficient and minimize wait times.	• Patients will be informed of delays longer than 15 minutes. • Patients will be offered 24-hour dose of medicine. • Total visit time will be 60 minutes or less, including lab and radiology.

Reprinted, with permission, 1997 from Saint Mary's Hospital, Green Bay, Wisconsin

4. Go one more step to make sure the standards are achievable. Ask your team, "What can we do to make sure we always meet these expectations?" Debug your processes and revamp them as needed so that everyone knows how they can reliably meet your standards.

Tips

• Use benchmarking to set standards. Call other services and investigate to find out whether they have service standards in place. Compare yours to theirs and see what levels of performance you want to set. This can give you a reality check on what are achievable levels. Also, you might want to decide to aim higher than they do to meet expectations important to customers, in order to gain a competitive advantage.

• Make sure you involve staff in the standard-setting process so that you don't end up with a list of pie-in-the-sky standards that staff resent because systems problems or other barriers block them from achieving these standards.

Step 7: Set Service Targets

As a result of listening to what your customers say they care about, you'll probably establish many service standards, after agreeing on achievable levels of service. But to gain a competitive advantage over other services and to achieve a level of impressive service for your customers' top priorities, consider also setting service targets— a small number of stretch goals that, when reached, will have a significant impact on customer satisfaction and can become standards. Targets are stretch goals for raising a particular standard even higher. For instance, if your standard has been to give people an appointment time that is no longer than two weeks from their call date, how much difference would it make to them if you gave them an appointment within one week, not two? If you could achieve this, would it set you apart from your competitors? That's the kind of discussion you need to have, first with customers and then with staff, to identify service targets.

You can also set service targets by looking at your satisfaction data and selecting targets for those service features your customers want that they don't currently rate high. Here are data from a satisfaction survey Saint Mary's Hospital uses to monitor performance related to several of their service standards that customers selected as key to their satisfaction. They took the results and listed them from high satisfaction to low satisfaction (in Pareto chart order). They then focused on the ones at the bottom, setting stretch goals so that staff would work together to figure out how to raise the standards.

First Care Customer Expectations

Expectation	Mean Score (in Pareto chart order)
Convenient hours	6.91
24-hour dose of prescriptions if needed	6.84
Billing your insurance company	6.75
Having a quality, competent staff.	6.66
Keeping patients informed	6.41
Providing a sense of being separate from the emergency department	6.12
Short waiting times	6.02

Source: Saint Mary's Hospital, Green Bay, Wisconsin, 1997

Be sure to engage staff in the process of setting service targets.

 Stretch Goals

This tool will help you to engage staff in setting stretch goals in the form of service targets.

Method

1. Convene staff or a representative group.
2. Show recent customer feedback, including information collected earlier about what's most important to customers.
3. Invite answers to this question: "To impress our customers, where should we aim to raise our standards?" List the responses.
4. Now, give everyone two votes. Have them vote for two of the possible stretch goals by applying this criterion: "What would

matter most to our customers while also being achievable if we set our collective minds to it?"

5. After agreeing on one of them, identify barriers in the way of raising performance. Subdivide people into miniteams to tackle these barriers and see if they can reduce them—removing the current ceiling on performance related to that standard.

Tips

- This can be exciting if you let the stretch goals come from staff, instead of imposing them. Leave genuine room for staff ownership! Engage staff in setting stretch targets, so that they feel an investment in figuring out how to reach them and so that they take pride in their achievement.
- Feel free to give your own opinions of appropriate stretch targets, but don't insist unless there is a compelling reason from customers for setting a particular target.
- Check your targets with customers. Ask, "What would you think if we could deliver this to you?" Make sure your targets make a difference to customers.
- Hold problem-solving, barrier removal, or process improvement team meetings in order to figure out what's blocking service performance from reaching the targets. Focus staff on debugging your systems and people's behavior so that stretch goals become achievable, not frustratingly out of reach.

Step 8: Monitor Performance

Needless to say, you need to monitor service performance related to your standards and targets. Otherwise, you won't know how you're doing, and all that work you devoted to developing standards might be to no avail. The big benefit of instituting monitors—simple monitors—is that you can give results to staff. Feedback is the most powerful booster of service improvement that there is. It's simple.

You have identified staff behaviors key to customers. You translated these behaviors into job-specific behaviors using protocols and scripts. So, staff know exactly what they need to do to meet customer expectations. You crystallized standards so everyone knows the goals you're trying to meet in a measurable way. When you measure how you're doing, everyone not only can feel good about positive results, but also every staff member can see the direct result of their personal contribution to living up to the standard and to the customer satisfaction level that resulted.

The same is true for disappointing feedback. If you monitor service performance in relation to standards and targets, you can let people know when performance fails to hit the mark, and this tends to spur on good, well-intentioned people to try to hit the mark next time. Here are some examples:

Standard	Measure
Written results to referring physician within 24 hours	Person who mails/faxes results reports keeps log of test date, date results arrive, and date sent.
100% of patients will be discharged with written results.	Discharge checklist includes written results received by patient to take home.
Patients will be contacted every 15 minutes of wait time.	Registrar has log for arrival time, contact time (#1, #2, #3, and so on), and time taken.
Total visit time 60 minutes or less, including lab/radiology	Departure time on log mentioned above
100% of patients will receive follow-up call, including weekends within 48-hour time frame	Patient follow-up checklist includes follow-up phone call, date _____, time _____ by _____

Logs, checklists, observation tools, surveys, and other measurement devices are all possibilities for tracking performance in relation to standards.

Monitor Design

This tool will assist you in identifying a measuring method you can use to track performance related to each standard.

Method
There's no trick to this. Just try this straightforward approach:

1. Bring staff together. Challenge them to help you develop a simple measuring device for each standard.
2. Focus on one standard at a time.
   —Brainstorm alternative ways to measure performance related to that standard.
   —Vote for the one that seems most promising (it reflects the seedling of a good idea).
3. Take the winners (those voted most promising) and ask staff to try to make each one simple and easy to use.
4. See if you can reach agreement.
5. With the same people, work out who can collect and manage the data for each standard. Work out your plans so the measurement actually happens.
6. Post the measures on a huge bulletin board as our report card, to remind people of what you're measuring.
7. Measure.
8. Inform the staff of the results in a meeting, on a bulletin board, in a memo, or some combination of these.

Tips

- Don't let the potential tedium of data collection stop you from developing and using monitors. Monitors are critical because without them, you might have standards but no accountability. Monitors enable your team to answer the question, "Are we living up to our standards? Are we keeping our promises to our customers?"
- If you focus on finding simple methods, you will. There are simple methods that consume minimal staff time and that require no research expertise.
- You probably have one or two people on your team particularly good at this because of their cognitive style. Ask them to be the standards monitor subcommittee and do the lion's share of the design work.

Step 9: Hold Yourself and Your Team Accountable

Expectations are all clear now—including expectations for staff behavior, protocols for steps along your customers' pathways through your services, and commitments you're willing to make to customers in the form of your standards. That's all well and good, but will you insist that you and staff live by these and enforce them? With service behaviors, protocols, scripts, standards, and targets, when push comes to shove, you, the manager, must hold staff accountable, creating consequences for people who persistently fail to follow these behavioral guidelines.

This step is for you, the manager. Hopefully, you will be able to engage staff in raising the standards and living up to them. But there might be some individuals who just don't live up to the standards. It is ultimately your job to coach them, to confront them about their behavior, and if they don't take your coaching and feedback seriously or can't meet the standard despite their best efforts, to terminate their employment. If you are ultimately unwilling to do this, others on your team see that the standards are options, not requirements, and they don't work quite so hard to uphold them. Everyone loses: you, your customers, and your team.

Tried-and-True Model for Confronting Service Performance Problems by Staff

When you see staff members who violate your standards or fail to use the protocols that they know they're supposed to use, confront them about the behavior or they might think their behavior is acceptable as is. Here is a great format for providing feedback to employees whose service performance violates standards.

Method

When confronting a team member who violates the standard or doesn't use the protocol, take the following steps:

1. State your positive intention. For example, a manager says to a staff member, "I want to talk with you about my observations of your behavior since I know you care about our customers."
2. Describe the problematic behavior. For example, a manager says to the staff member, "When Mr. Sidney came in, you said hello in a curt manner and with a lifeless voice. You did not call him by name even though you've seen him many times and

have his name right there in the appointment book. And you did not remind him of who you are."

3. Explain the consequences of the problematic behavior for customers and/or for your service. For example, a manager says to a staff member, "This behavior is a problem because it makes the patient feel unwelcome and uncomfortable. It reflects on all of us because, from the patient's point of view, we seem to find it acceptable to act in a disinterested fashion. And it affects the future of our service by creating a dissatisfied customer who might not return to us for service and certainly is unlikely to tell their friends anything good about us."

4. Let the team member talk. Listen and show you understand what he or she is saying.

5. Express a pinch of empathy. Since health care staff tend to be caring, idealistic people, few treat customers poorly intentionally. Sometimes there are pressures that make it difficult for employees to be as good as they know how to be. By expressing a pinch of empathy, you acknowledge that other pressures might be making it hard to be service oriented. For example, a manager says to staff, "I realize that this has been a very hectic day for you and that you've been running ragged."

6. Relating the behavior to the standard or protocol, state the behavior you expect in the future in no uncertain terms. For example, "We put a lot of work into developing protocols for people to use with their customers when they greet them. Despite the pressures on you, from now on, I expect you to greet each patient warmly, quickly, with a smile, and by name."

7. Check back with the team member the next day to see how he or she is doing and to discuss any loose ends or questions.

 Tips

- Use the same model to confront your team if many people seem to be letting the standards slip.
- Remember to keep your feedback specific, behavioral, and to the point.
- When you see problem behavior, give staff feedback and coach them, in hopes that they will do better. Usually, they do change their behavior as a result. If they don't, escalate your approach

still further. Counsel them again and support their efforts to change. If they don't, give them a warning and troubleshoot with them what's in the way of improvement. After you've given them considerable feedback and support, if they haven't changed their behavior, terminate their employment. Otherwise, your service standards collapse as other staff members realize they have been built on a weak foundation, namely your willingness to tolerate less.

Conclusion

Setting standards and making them stick is just about the most difficult challenge in creating and sustaining impressive service. Many service managers pontificate about the importance of giving great service but stop short of helping staff define what that exactly means. By taking the time and care with your team to define service behaviors, job-specific protocols and scripts, service standards, and targets, you translate a vague vision of impressive service into a concrete picture of what impressive service really requires.

This takes you a great distance, but it still isn't enough. You need to hold yourself, your team, and every individual accountable for upholding the standards and using the protocols effectively by installing measures of performance and by confronting problematic performance when you become aware of it. Prepare yourself to go to the limit with accountability if you're serious about achieving high standards of employee behavior.

If you want phenomenal breakthroughs, go for the gusto in the area of standards and accountability. Persistence and commitment to this area, in all of its facets, is the closest thing you'll find to a magic bullet for building and maintaining a consistently impressive service.

Notes

1. Adapted, with permission, from Gail Scott and Associates © 1997.

2. Ibid.

Chapter 3

• • •

Help Staff Hear the Voice of the Customer

Do You Need to Read This Chapter?

- Do your staff have hectic workloads and rush from person to person and task to task?
- Do staff feel insecure about their own futures, and are they much more absorbed with their own feelings than those of their customers?
- Do your staff feel oppressed by the tumultuous changes going on in health care that affect them and as a result seem resentful and unsettled?
- Have some staff been doing the same job for years, causing their jobs to become routine and their approach robotic?
- Are you under so much pressure to reach financial goals that quality and patient satisfaction goals have taken a backseat?

If you answered yes to even one of these questions, your team runs the risk of not being tuned in to your customers' voices. Your staff might have closed their ears to people's concerns, needs, feelings, and suggestions.

Not many people want to hear this. Employees think more like this:

- If I listen, I'll hear about more of their needs, and I can't even meet those I know about now.
- It just frustrates me to hear customer needs, because I can't give them what they want, and I feel like a failure.

- Who has time to listen?!
- The only important customer these days is the payer. The patient be damned. So that's where our heads have to be!
- The good old days are over. Patients can't expect what they used to get. And I don't want to *hear* how I'm disappointing them.
- I'm just too busy, and, anyway, I already know what customers want and need.

But these days, it's not that easy for you or your staff to stay tuned in to customers' needs and feelings. If you're under great pressure to attract business and reach financial goals in this hotly competitive marketplace, your head is likely to be on the business, much more than on the people. If your staff feel overworked, scattered, and unsettled about their futures, they become intensely task oriented or self-absorbed.

The net result is that the customer's voice becomes dim, if not inaudible. In your efforts to handle your work volume and meet financial goals, you and your team might have closed your ears to your customers.

This Is a Crisis

When we drown out our customers' voices with our own concerns and goals, the customer feels lost, ignored, and neglected. When we close ourselves off to the voice of the customer, we lose the hands-down most powerful way to stay on course. Customer feedback helps us target our efforts and make course corrections. Also, when we stop listening to customers, we miss the chance to get their reactions to new ideas and possibilities for meeting or exceeding their expectations.

You no doubt agree that most people in health care want to do right by patients. Most recognize that health care customers are vulnerable. They worry. They hurt. And many have feelings of fear and powerlessness in the face of health care providers. When staff members tune in to these feelings, they are likely to do right by customers. They listen. They're gentle. They protect privacy. They communicate respectfully, and in many, many ways, they show their care and compassion for customers' feelings and needs. It's when staff are *not* tuned in to customers that the insensitivity and problems occur.

If all of this resonates with you and you admit that your customers' voices are not ringing loud and clear throughout your service, read on and you'll find very powerful methods of restoring and strengthening the voice of the customer in your service.

In this chapter, we present three kinds of tools to help you and your staff tune in to customer concerns:

1. Tools to help you channel customer feedback directly to your staff
2. Tools to help staff adopt the perspective of customers and see their services through their customers' eyes
3. Tools to show your staff how to maintain an awareness of their customers' perspectives in their everyday work and decisions

Channeling Customer Feedback Directly to Your Staff

Often, when a manager tells staff what customers want, staff feel resentful. They feel lectured to, even patronized. It's different and much more powerful when they hear from their customers directly. When customers express themselves to staff, their feelings and perceptions feel like facts, unfiltered by you and what you want staff to do about them. When staff hear from customers directly, they are much more likely to take the feedback to heart and adjust their attention and performance in the direction of better satisfying their customers.

In the following subsections, we explain three tools that turn up the volume on customers' voices:

1. The success indicators process
2. Staff as pulse takers
3. Homegrown focus groups

The Success Indicators Process[1]

Success indicators are a quick and easy way to get real-time feedback about what is and isn't working for customers. With an inherent desire to do good for customers, such feedback has the power to keep our attention on customer needs and concerns.

1. Heartfelt thanks to Lynda Rothman, senior consultant with Gail Scott and Associates, for this wonderful tool.

Why do you need success indicators? Good question. Here are some answers:

- To identify the particular needs and concerns of each major customer group
- To be able to assess quickly and accurately the impact of service improvements from customers' points of view; to know what is working and what needs to be improved
- To speed up the feedback cycle, so you get customer input from patients, physicians, and employees quickly
- To have an easy mechanism for getting candid feedback from customers
- To supplement anecdotal feedback with quantitative data so you have a more complete picture of your service quality
- To have a systematic way to find problems when you're implementing service improvements

There are so many good reasons to institute a system of success indicators, but if you're human and in health care, you probably want to scream, "How can I possibly do one more thing!!!!!" Take a breath and relax. Although design and installation of success indicators do require work up front and ongoing data collection, you can keep the process simple. You will be so glad to have concrete customer feedback that the benefits more than compensate for the anxiety and work involved.

The Success Indicators Process in Five Steps
By going through the following five steps, you can institute relevant success indicators, track results related to these indicators, and use the results to trigger both recognition of successes and pursuit of improvement opportunities.

The Success Indicators Process in Five Steps

1. Identify your service's key customers.
2. Ask customers what's important to them in terms of service in order to identify four success indicator questions per customer group.
3. Collect baseline data.
4. Collect data at frequent intervals.
5. Use the data to celebrate success and to guide course corrections.

Let's say you have a cardiac surgery service. You identify three key customer groups that concern you most: patients, their families, and referring physicians. Ask each customer group what's important to them in terms of service—in order to identify four success indicator questions per customer group.

From surveys and discussion with patients, you learn that, most importantly, patients want the following:

- Staff who do everything possible to relieve the stress of surgery
- To know what to expect at every point in the process
- To trust the responsiveness of their caregivers
- To feel that their care is well coordinated, that one hand knows what the other hand is doing

From surveys and discussion with the patient's family members, you learn that, foremost, they want the following:

- Staff to volunteer information about the patient's status and follow-up needs
- Staff to welcome their questions
- Staff responsiveness to their loved one's needs
- Staff who respect them for their key role in supporting the patient

From surveys and discussions with referring physicians, you learn that referring physicians most want

- To be kept up to date about their patients
- To be communicated with in a timely manner by the surgery team
- To be consulted at choice points in the patient's care
- To hear from their patients that they are satisfied with their care

Based on this upfront work, you and/or a team develop success indicator report cards specific to each customer group.

Patients: How Are We Doing?

Please help us to improve our services by answering these four questions.

1. How would you evaluate the steps staff took to prevent or relieve the stress and anxiety surrounding your surgery?
    _____ Disappointing
    _____ Adequate
    _____ Good
    _____ Impressive

2. How well did staff keep you informed about what to expect at every point in your experience with us?
    _____ Poor
    _____ Fair
    _____ Good
    _____ Impressive

3. How responsive have staff been when you've needed them for any reason?
    _____ Very unresponsive
    _____ Somewhat unresponsive
    _____ Somewhat responsive
    _____ Very responsive

4. How well do you think your care was coordinated?
    _____ Poor
    _____ Fair
    _____ Good
    _____ Impressive

Please provide any comments or suggestions related to our care or service.

Please leave your survey on your meal tray or ask any staff or family member to drop it into the survey box at the nurses' station.
Thank you.

Family Members: How Are We Doing?

Please help us to improve our services by answering these four questions about our care and services.

1. How effective have caregivers been in keeping you informed about your loved one's status?
   _____ Very ineffective
   _____ Somewhat ineffective
   _____ Somewhat effective
   _____ Impressive

2. To what extent have staff welcomed your questions and concerns?
   _____ Hardly at all
   _____ To a moderate extent
   _____ To a considerable extent
   _____ It's been impressive

3. How responsive have staff been to your loved one's needs?
   _____ Very unresponsive
   _____ Somewhat unresponsive
   _____ Somewhat responsive
   _____ Very responsive

4. How respectful have staff been to you about your key role in the patient's care and healing?
   _____ Hardly respectful at all
   _____ Somewhat disrespectful
   _____ Somewhat respectful
   _____ It's been impressive

Please provide any comments or suggestions related to our care or service.

Please leave your survey on a meal tray or drop it into the survey box at the nurses' station.
Thank you.

To Physicians Who Referred Patients for Cardiac Surgery: How Are We Doing?

Please help us to improve our cardiac surgery services by answering these four questions.

1. How well have you been kept up to date about your patient's status?
    _____ Very poorly
    _____ Somewhat poorly
    _____ Somewhat well
    _____ Very well

2. How courteously have you been treated when you visit or make inquiries?
    _____ Not at all courteously
    _____ Somewhat discourteously
    _____ Somewhat courteously
    _____ It's been impressive

3. Have you been consulted at choice points in the patient's care?
    _____ No
    _____ Sometimes
    _____ Regularly

4. In the last 12 months, how satisfied have your patients been with the care and service they've received in our cardiac surgery service?
    _____ Very dissatisfied
    _____ Somewhat dissatisfied
    _____ Somewhat satisfied
    _____ Impressed

Please provide any comments or suggestions related to our care or service.

Return your completed survey in this postage-paid mailer.
Thank you very much.

These feedback forms don't need to be elaborate or fancy or technically sophisticated. They need to make sense to staff and be developed with staff involvement.

Here's another example from a medical practice. This medical practice had a history of complaints and frustrations associated with an obsolete manual scheduling system for patient appointments. As a result of patient, staff, and physician complaints, they installed a new scheduling system and developed success indicators to track the results related to key indicators relevant to each customer group's concerns. This example shows how you can use the success indicators process to track results of a change or improvement in service.

Before implementing the dramatically different scheduling system, a planning team consulted patients and doctors to find out what they wanted. Patients desired the following:

- To get an appointment in a timely fashion
- To be treated courteously by the person who answers the phone
- To be taken on time when they arrive for their appointment
- To be offered a convenient appointment time

Physicians said that they wanted the following:

- To optimize use of their time, having neither too many, nor too few patients during their work hours
- To avoid complaints from patients about their accessibility
- To work with office staff who are able to handle the scheduling system autonomously
- To avoid keeping patients waiting too long once they arrive for their appointments

Staff wanted the following:

- To have a user-friendly system
- To reduce patient complaints about access to appointments
- To reduce waiting times for patient
- To make it possible to make changes in appointments easily

A team of staff developed these success indicator report cards as a result.

Patients: How Are We Doing with Scheduling?

Please help us to evaluate our scheduling system by answering four questions.

1. When you called for an appointment, how many days/weeks did you have to wait before the appointment?
   _____ Too long
   _____ A reasonable length of time
   _____ Not long at all

2. Regarding time of day and day of the week, how easy or hard was it to get an appointment time convenient for you?
   _____ Very hard
   _____ So-so
   _____ Very easy

3. When you called for an appointment, how courteous was the person who handled your call?
   _____ Not courteous
   _____ Moderately courteous
   _____ Very courteous

4. When you arrived for your appointment, how long did you have to wait to see the doctor?
   _____ 30 minutes or more
   _____ 15 to 30 minutes
   _____ Less than 15 minutes

Please provide any comments or suggestions related to our scheduling system:

Please drop your survey into the survey box at the front desk.
Thank you!

Physicians: How Are We Doing with Scheduling?

Please help us to evaluate our scheduling system by answering four questions.

1. How well is our scheduling system optimizing your time, so that you have neither too few nor too many patients during your work hours?
   ____ Not well at all
   ____ So-so
   ____ Very well

2. In the last month, how often have patients complained to you about problems they had getting appointments?
   ____ Seldom
   ____ A moderate number of times
   ____ Often

3. Over the last month, how often have staff involved you with problems or special needs related to patient scheduling?
   ____ Seldom
   ____ A moderate amount of times
   ____ Often

4. In the last month, how often did you find yourself keeping patients waiting too long?
   ____ Very often
   ____ A moderate amount of time
   ____ Rarely

Please provide any comments or suggestions related to our scheduling system.

Please drop your survey into the survey box at the front desk.
Thank you!

Staff: How Are We Doing with Scheduling?

Please help us to evaluate our scheduling system by answering four questions.

1. How easy is it to use our scheduling system?
   _____ Hard
   _____ So-so
   _____ Easy

2. How frequently do patients complain about access to appointments?
   _____ Very frequently
   _____ Moderately frequent
   _____ Infrequently

3. Generally, how long do patients have to wait once they arrive for their appointments?
   _____ A long time
   _____ A moderate amount of time
   _____ A very short time

4. How easy or hard is it to make changes in people's appointments using our scheduling system?
   _____ Hard
   _____ So-so
   _____ Easy

Please provide any comments or suggestions related to our scheduling system.

Please drop your survey into the survey box at the front desk.
Thank you!

For both examples, with their report cards in hand, staff developed and implemented a system for collecting baseline data and a regular schedule of ongoing data collection. They processed the data monthly. Then, within two days of processing it, they posted it and discussed it at a staff meeting where the team acknowledged successes and improvements and also targeted opportunities for further improvement.

How to Complete Each Step in the Success Indicators Process

1. Identify your service's key customers.
   —For most services, the key customer groups are patients and their families, employees, physicians, payers, and referral sources. Pinpoint yours.
   —Prepare a preliminary list of key customers, then make sure that key leaders agree with your list.
2. Ask customers what's important in order to identify four questions (success indicators) per customer group. (*Note:* Limit the number of questions you'll ultimately ask each customer group. Most organizations, services, and practices make four the magic number because this number forces them to select the vital few questions they're committed to acting on! In addition, use a strategy appropriate for each customer group to find out what's most important to them.)
   —Consult patients
     –Create a list of 10 to 15 items that you think may be important to patients and create a "what's important" form. The form asks patients to select the three items most important to them.
     –Survey 25 percent of the patients or 20 patients (whichever is greater) during a one-week period.
   —Consult physicians
     –Use a similar process to that for patients. Also, consider supplementing it with some discussion with physicians, so that you more fully understand their concerns.
     –Try to survey at least 70 percent of the physicians active in your area. Also, tell physicians you'll follow up frequently with a simple survey.
   —Consult employees
     –Ideally, hold a meeting with all employees to engage them and build their commitment. Try to get 100 percent participation.
     –Have the employees brainstorm a list of what's important and then multivote to select the most important items. (In multivoting, each person gets multiple votes that they can allocate. For example, if they have five votes, they can give all five to one item, or four to one item and one to a different item, or one vote to each of five different items, and so on.)
3. Collect baseline data. Baseline data are important so that you know whether changes have occurred over time. In the ideal

world, you would collect baseline data over an extended period. In the real world, you need enough data so that, in your judgment, the baseline data reflect the current reality for your various customers.

—Create a survey box for each unit/service's data.

—Color-code the surveys for different customer types to make them easy to sort.

—We suggest one week for all baseline data collection.

–Patient data: Survey 100 percent of the patients on three different days during one week (for instance, in a hospital, the day shift on Tuesday, the evening shift on Thursday, and the day shift on Saturday). This provides feedback from weekdays and weekends as well as from different shifts.

–Employee data: Distribute employee surveys to all staff with the requirement that they turn them in during the designated baseline week.

–Physician data: Try to survey at least 70 percent of the key physicians as they are available during the designated week.

4. Collect data at frequent intervals.

—Watch your time intervals.

–Collect data as frequently as you can so that you can look at not just data points representing a particular day but also trends over time. The goal is to capture a picture of what is and is not working for the various customer groups on a given day, so you can identify problems and begin to know what to improve. You need to find a way to process the data very quickly, make it available, and trigger actions.

–Gather data every 5th day for the first 30 days after implementation. After the first 30 days, gather data every 12th day for three cycles. Then, repeat the data collection at 6- and 12-month intervals after implementation for comparison.

—Keep your methods simple. To keep the time involved to a minimum, make sure your surveys are simple to complete and simple to analyze. The survey needs to include the following:

–A brief statement about your commitment to improvement and customer satisfaction

–Simple, clear instructions

–Success indicators and an answer scale, along with space for comments

–Questions regarding what else the organization can do to meet their needs (especially for patients and physicians)

–A thank-you for participating

–Instructions on what to do with the completed form.

—Clearly define whom to survey. For instance, survey the following:

–All employees who work during a designated 24-hour period

–All physicians who physically come on to the unit/service during that time

–All patients who are admitted for more then four hours. (Alternate between days and nights for patient surveys.)

—Process and post the data on the unit/service within 24 hours of the end of the survey period. This is key! Since you are only asking four questions of each customer group, this is doable if you set your mind to it. The posted data should include the following:

–The average score for each item for this time period

–A trend chart that also includes the baseline data

–Written comments, along with specific names of staff members if the comments are positive. If a staff member's name is associated with a negative comment, give the name to the manager instead of posting it.

–Plenty of room for recording action steps on the data display

—Post the data where employees and physicians, but not patients, can see it.

5. Use the data to celebrate success and guide course corrections.

—Use the data in a variety of ways:

–Celebrate the positive findings.

–Sort the data and comments that reflect opportunities for improvement into priority order and develop action plans.

–Use the data as a trigger to solicit further anecdotal feedback from employees and physicians. For example, if a physician says that a change is just not working, locate him or her and invite examples and discussion. This will also help if a problem is an isolated instance (special cause) or reflects a pattern in need of a process change.

–If you gather data in another way for some of the same customer groups (for example, physician or patient satisfaction surveys), compare your data with this other data over time.

—Focus people on the data:

–Staff: Plan for a brief employee meeting on the day you post the new data. At that meeting, celebrate the successes (with food!). Engage staff in helping to set priorities for improvement and developing action plans.

–Physicians: Set aside time to connect with key physicians to share the data and written comments and also, most importantly, your action plans. Solicit their reactions and further input.

A Short Pep Talk

If you're wondering if you can afford to institute success indicators because of the time and effort involved, change the question to its opposite. Can you afford not to institute success indicators?

Data and feedback are really important to improving service quality in a purposeful, rational way. But our health care industry hasn't done a very good job of figuring out the data we need and how to get it easily. Also problematic is how to use the data once it's collected and how to involve frontline people in the process, so that their sense of ownership translates into active use of the information.

You have a chance to make a real difference by instituting success indicators. And it's doable. Your staff will see that the resulting feedback is truly helpful and the collection process doesn't have to be overwhelming. They'll also be inspired to stick with your change process because feedback from success indicators gives people instant positive reinforcement directly from their customers, and this keeps caring health care professionals going.

Adapt the success indicators process in whatever way makes sense for your service or organization. The goal is to institute a simple, fast, reliable, and manageable way to listen to your customers, and use their voices to guide staff in making improvements in your services.

 Staff as Pulse Takers

Here's another way to involve staff in soliciting feedback so that it's channeled directly from customers to staff. This tool has two purposes:

1. To engage staff in collecting feedback directly from customers, so that they can feel good about what's working
2. To share customer needs and concerns with coworkers in a team effort to improve service

You can use either formal or informal methods.

- A formal approach: Set the expectation that every staff member interviews two patients a week about their experience with the service and feeds the results back to all staff. Instead of having to go through hoops assigning patients, assign each staff member a time period during which they need to interview two patients. If the time periods do not overlap, then staff will not run the risk of approaching the same patient more than once.
- An informal approach: Get staff so interested in customer feedback that they think to ask for feedback throughout their work. AT&T has created a ritual way of doing this that has impressed customers. When you call customer service at AT&T, the person ends the interaction with the question, "Are you satisfied with the outcome of this call?" At this point, the operator gets feedback (and so might any supervisor who might be listening in).

Method

1. Imagine the great feedback available to staff if, at the end of every service, they asked:
   —How satisfied are you with your services here today?
   —What complaints or concerns do you have at this point?
   —What suggestions do you have about how we could have improved your experience with us?
2. Or how about these three questions:
   —How did we do today?
   —What else could we help you with?
   —What should I know about the service given by our team?
3. Staff can also take the pulse by conducting telephone interviews one to three days after a person has been served by your service. This can double as a way to follow up on the patient's condition and, at the same time, invite comments about satisfaction and complaints related to the service received.
   —Consider this for a medical practice. Some physicians have the office manager or nurse conduct these interviews. Others have all staff (including the physicians) conduct a few interviews, getting everyone involved and developing a stake in patient satisfaction. For example, Dr. Hill has a group practice with 10 other physicians. Dr. Hill, her office manager, and their receptionist develop the interview. Dr. Hill holds

training for all staff and shares her belief that the future of their practice rests on happy patients. She asks every person in the practice to get involved in getting patient feedback during the last week of every month. Specifically, she says she wants to assign four patients to each staff member and have the staff member call these patients on the phone to ask about their experiences with the practice. Dr. Hill hands out a list of the questions that her committee developed. She divides people into pairs and asks them to try the questions on one another. Afterward, the group refines the questions and discusses ways to handle people who don't seem to have much to say, and so on.

Medical Practice: Phone Interview with Patients

Hello, this is _____ from Dr. _____'s office. How are you feeling? [Listen and be responsive. Then, move on.] I wanted to know how you're doing, and I also have another reason for calling. Several of us from our office are calling patients who visited our office during the last month to ask a few questions about how they viewed their experience with our practice. We're trying to make changes in our practice in order to give our patients the service they deserve. I'd like to know if you would be willing to answer a few questions about your experience with us. I'd like to arrange for a five-minute, confidential interview with you at a time convenient for you—now or at a more convenient time. Would you agree to that? Great! I really appreciate your taking the time. Let me begin . . .

1. What did you like about your last visit to our office?
2. What bothered you about your last visit to our office? Please feel free to mention anything big or small, since that will help us make things better.
3. What can we do to make our service better for you?

[Push here for many suggestions, a wish list.]

Closing: Mrs./Mr./Ms. _____, I really appreciate your willingness to answer these questions so frankly. It helps us know what we're doing right and what we need to work on in order to give you the quality of service you deserve. Thanks so much, and I hope you feel better/continue to feel better/continue to feel well.

4. Use pulse taking with your different customer groups—for instance, family members or companions of your patients—and also referral sources. Many people go to medical appointments with a friend or family member, and visitors visit patients in hospitals. Companions often go into exam or procedure rooms or consulting rooms along with the patient. Other times, the companion sits and waits in a waiting area. In both cases, this observer sees a lot about your service. Feeling protective of and concerned about their loved ones, they scrutinize what's happening and see it all. They tend to be keenly astute because of their inclination to be advocates for their loved one's welfare.

—Use while-you-wait interviews to take advantage of the time they spend sitting around watching. Invite their perceptions and suggestions, and at the same time, by occupying them, you'll make their time go faster. You're also communicating the message that you think they're important, not invisible.

—Tap into their views by having a member of your staff sit down with them for a few minutes and ask a few questions. A survey might look like this:

Interview Your Patient's Family or Companion

Here you sit . . . waiting. While you're waiting, you have a chance to see how we function here, and you know how our office and people make you feel. Would you be willing to share your opinions of this medical practice, based on your own observations and anything you might have heard about us before? I'll keep your views confidential. I'm really hoping you'll be frank and not be concerned about anyone here knowing who said what!

[After getting their consent]

1. What do you like about this medical practice, if anything (environment, staff, doctors, getting here, waiting area, other facilities, and so on)?
2. What don't you like about this practice [same probes as above]?
3. What would you change here in order to make this the ideal medical practice?

Thank you very much for helping us, and I hope all goes well for your friend or loved one.

—Similar questions can be asked of people by office staff. Or, you can identify specific questions about aspects of your practice you particularly want to learn more about. An example follows.

Survey for a Patient's Family or Companion

Here you sit, waiting for your friend or family member. Would you be willing to share your views about the experience you're having in our waiting room? It will help us make future waits more tolerable.

1. Regarding the physical environment in this waiting area, how do you feel about the following:
   —The colors you see
   —Furniture arrangement
   —Chair comfort
   —Sounds you hear
   —Air temperature
   —Things available to do to make the time go faster
   —Staff behavior toward you
2. Please share any suggestions or ideas you have about how we can make the experience of waiting here more pleasant.
   —Any amenities or conveniences we could provide
   —Environmental improvements
   —Other suggestions

5. If your service receives referrals from other physicians, community agencies, or other professional groups, ask them for feedback about what they see and what they hear secondhand about your services. Referral sources are, after all, customers whose referrals help build your business and reputation. Have staff make quarterly calls to a selection of referrers. Ask questions like these:

Tap Referral Source Perceptions

1. What have you heard about our service/practice?
2. What have you heard about our positive features?
3. What have you heard about our weaknesses or negative aspects?
4. How do you feel about our relationship with you as a valued referrer?
   —How well do we communicate with you?

—How can we communicate better?

—Do we refer patients back to you at the appropriate point in their treatment?

—What suggestions do you have about how we can improve our communication with you?

5. What suggestions do you have for making our practice/service more responsive to you and the people you tend to refer?

6. Simple questions and simple surveys like these can be used to gather great feedback in a whole host of situations, too. Help staff identify the diverse opportunities they have to interview people, for instance:

—They can ask a few questions of customers right after they register for service while they're waiting. They can interview people about the welcome they got, their ease or difficulty finding their way, their experience getting the appointment, their comfort in the office, and the nature of any anxiety they might feel right then that staff might ease.

—They can interview a customer's companion about his or her perceptions of the service.

—They can interview customers right after their appointment— while they're getting their coat or after they arrive home or the next day.

—They can ask questions while the customer is waiting for a prescription, test result, or another piece of information.

There are no doubt many other opportunities that your staff can identify.

7. Make it easy for staff at first by assigning questions and respondents to them. Later, staff efforts to solicit feedback will be more informal. They'll ask questions like these automatically once they realize the value of hearing the voices of their customers.

8. Make it easier for staff by building their skill. Getting staff to be effective as feedback solicitors isn't as easy as it sounds because many, if not most, staff have trouble inviting direct face-to-face feedback in an open, nondefensive manner. They also have trouble reporting back the results objectively. Help them develop the skills and comfort they need. Help your staff build skill in asking open-ended questions in a nondefensive manner

and listening to the customer without interpreting or modifying what they hear to meet or soothe their own needs. Here is a round-robin meeting design that helps to build such skills.

Round-Robin Practice for Staff Pulse Takers

First, give a short pitch on the importance of asking open-ended, not leading, questions, and also listening thoroughly without defensiveness.

Then, divide your team into trios, called person A, B, and C. In round 1, have person A play staff pulse taker, person B play patient, and person C play observer.

1. Provide pulse takers with a short list of questions. Start with these and invite the whole group to refine the list and make it manageable.
   —How satisfied are you with your services here today?
   —What complaints or concerns do you have at this point?
   —What suggestions do you have about how we could have improved your experience with us?
2. Ask pulse takers to approach person B—the patient—to do the following:
   —Explain their desire to get feedback from the patient about their experience and ask their willingness to participate
   —Ask the questions, listen carefully, and probe for further information
   —End the interaction with a statement of appreciation for the patient's candor and thoughtfulness
3. Challenge the pulse takers to do this questioning with the following style:
   —Listening and thoroughly hearing the patient out
   —Avoiding any defensiveness whatsoever
   —Avoiding explaining or lecturing or discounting anything the patient says
   —And showing throughout an interest in what the patient has to say and an appreciation that the patient is speaking up
4. Also, ask the pulse takers to take notes on what the patient said, with an eye to accurately reflecting it and not interpreting or in any way losing the patient's meaning.

Observers watch the practice session in which the pulse taker interviews the patient. Afterward,

5. The patient shares their feelings and perceptions of the process, including the following:
   —How did they feel being interviewed?
   —What did the pulse taker do to encourage openness and candor?
   —How well did the pulse taker listen and avoid getting defensive?
6. The observer shares their perceptions of how well the pulse taker did the following:
   —Introduced the purpose to the patient
   —Asked open-ended questions with appropriate probes to dig deeper
   —Encouraged the patient to speak, listened, and heard the patient out
   —Avoided showing any defensiveness, by not cutting the patient short, lecturing, or in any way discounting or explaining away anything the patient said
   —Showed interest and an appreciation that the patient was speaking up
   —Both patient and observer suggest ways the pulse taker could be more effective.

Then, the patient and observer examine the pulse taker's notes and give feedback on how objective these notes are, as opposed to interpreting or changing the patient's meaning or imposing the pulse taker's own attitudes and views.

After that, switch roles, so that person B becomes the pulse taker, person C becomes the patient, and so on. Go through the same process. Then switch roles again, so that all three people have a chance to practice being the pulse taker and getting feedback about his or her effectiveness.

Finally, have one pair role-play in front of the whole group, so that staff can see the model work one more time. This will help to cement the principles and skills involved and generate any further discussion needed. By the way, make sure you thank the pair that is willing to perform in front of everyone.

9. What can you do with the feedback? Make sure every staff person interviews at least three customers a month. Schedule a staff meeting once a month to share replies. Have staff interview their customers the week before so that patients' responses are fresh in their minds. At the staff meeting, discuss themes, identify improvement opportunities, and decide how to follow up. Ask the following:
    —What did you find out?
    —What surprised you?
    —What pleased you?
    —What are you inclined to want us to follow up on as a result?
10. And, of course, recognize people's efforts collecting the information.

Variations

- Begin staff meetings with the question, "What have you heard from customers about our service strengths and problems?" Bring in front desk staff and ask them what they've heard, too.
- Do ministudies that yield feedback about specific service improvements your team is pursuing. If you're working on improving access, focus for a month on access. Ask, "How accessible are we? What makes it easy? What makes it difficult to access us? What suggestions do you have about how we can improve your access to us?" If you're working on easing people's waiting time, ask about that. And so on.
- Alert staff to the need to get feedback from *all* customer groups. For instance, devote one month to interviewing referral sources or your payers to find out their perceptions of your services and their suggestions.
- Alternate the responsibility for pulse-taking interviews. For instance, have one person make 12 phone calls or do 12 in-person interviews a month, summarize the results, and report back to the staff at a monthly pulse-taking meeting. Then, engage another person.
- Hold a pizza dinner/lunch once a month after which people sit at phones (telethon style) and call patients. The next day, they have a protected, scheduled meeting at which they compare results and identify problems they want to solve in order to strengthen the service features of their practice.

Tips

- Use your influence as a role model. Let staff see you approaching customers and asking how their experience is. This is a far better way to improve service than scrutinizing staff behavior!
- Don't shortchange people on practice. Staff need help becoming comfortable asking for feedback and hearing it without defensiveness.
- Most important, emphasize with staff that inviting customer feedback and really listening to customers is probably the most powerful way to build positive relationships with customers and secure their loyalty. Even when customers aren't happy with your service, if you ask them to talk about their experience and if you listen well, they often end up impressed, not annoyed. They may even tell their friends and neighbors about your responsiveness. By listening to negatives as well as positives, you have a second chance to satisfy and impress customers and make things right.

Homegrown Focus Groups

Lots of health care organizations use focus groups to try out new service ideas, to test promotional campaigns, and to invite customer feedback. A focus group involves a small group in discussion to find out people's views about a certain subject. This tool for pulse taking involves the very powerful and efficient focus group technique, with a few unusual angles.

How does it work? A facilitator guides the discussion using a question guide. Focus groups work best when questions are open-ended and the facilitator encourages substantive discussion of each question within the group. Typical group size for a focus group is from 8 to 12 people, and most sessions take about 90 minutes.

In some organizations, a sponsor from the organization works with a professional focus group facilitator to develop the questions and facilitate the group. In other organizations, internal people conduct the focus groups themselves. In both cases, afterward, the facilitator and/or an invited coworker develops a report to summarize the findings, usually in written form, to the people seeking the information.

Without question, these kinds of focus groups are terrifically helpful because they solicit customer thoughts, feelings, and suggestions, and this provides a much better basis for decisions than a provider or producer perspective can in the absence of customer input. It's an efficient technique because you can learn from a whole group at a time. The group dynamics often lead to rich information because one person's thoughts trigger another person's memories and reactions.

These focus groups, however, often fall short of their full potential. Only a few people hear customers, and they're rarely the users of the feedback. Also, especially if you use professional focus group facilitators, data processors, and report writers, you're likely to sponsor few focus groups because of the expense involved.

The approach we recommend helps you get more out of customer focus groups by adding three elements:

1. Involve staff in generating the questions.
2. Instead of giving staff secondhand information, give them the much more powerful experience of actually attending the groups to see and hear customers talking firsthand. Too time consuming? Consider the benefits. Written reports lose a lot in the translation. The customers' own words are often missing, and certainly their facial expressions and body language are not captured. Staff hear what their customers are saying, and they will not think any sifting, sorting, or cleansing of information has been done by a data processor or manager before receiving the scoop. So, why disconnect staff from customer groups? Have them there, listening with their own ears and seeing their customers with their own eyes. The reality of their customers will hit home and influence their future actions and decisions. And if staff can't be there, get customers' permission to tape-record the discussion and pull staff together to listen to the tape.
3. Engage staff in sifting through the information to draw conclusions. Think of the last time that you read a list of someone else's conclusions from a research study. If you're typical, you think about the conclusions and whether you agree or not. If you're typical, you react with a low level of engagement because someone else processed the information and generated those conclusions. On the other hand, you are in a much more active mode if you gather the information and *you* sort through it and ask yourself, "What does this say to me?" You not only think about the end results, but you think and feel the information first. And you're much more invested in the conclusions.

Used correctly, this tool will give staff members powerful, first-hand information about customer thoughts and feelings and engage them in processing it and drawing conclusions from it—so that they are much more likely to use what they learn to guide their behavior and services.

Method

1. Identify someone who can facilitate your focus group. This person can be a professional focus group facilitator or an insider who has group dynamics skills, the ability to guide diverse people in discussion, and who can listen and probe without defensiveness (for example, a skilled social worker, educator, marketing person, patient relations person, human resources person, or the like). Engage this person in all planning, so that they get to know your team and the purpose of the group very, very well.

2. Convene staff to pinpoint the purpose of your focus group. Do you want to collect periodic feedback about your services? Are you seeking information from customers about a specific service challenge? Or, are you seeking reactions to an idea or proposal before instituting it (like a new service or a new service feature, or a new location, and so on)?

3. Talk with staff about who should be invited. Who exactly is the target group, and who is in a position to invite them to participate in a group?

4. Invite people to participate. A good approach is to write a letter of invitation and follow it up with a phone call.

Dear Ms. _____,

We are interested in making our patients' experiences with our medical practice as positive as possible.

On May 15th, [name of facilitator] will be holding a focus group dinner with several patients who use our practice. We invite you to be our guest at dinner. Also, we will provide you with a $25 honorarium to help cover your transportation, child care, or other expenses involved in attending this discussion. The purpose of the dinner is to invite people to share their views on our practice, its strengths, weaknesses, and how we can improve it to better satisfy our patients.

Will you join [name of facilitator] and several other patients for this dinner discussion?

Time: 7–9 p.m.
Place: Ming Garden

Please call my office at [phone number] to let me know if you can or cannot attend. I hope you can make it. If not, I want to encourage you to share your views and suggestions about our practice with any of our staff or me, so we can give you the quality of health care and service you deserve.

Thank you very much.

Sincerely,

[doctor's name], MD

5. Engage staff in developing the questions. To give you an idea of how intuitive and straightforward the questions can be, here's an example of a set of questions used in focus groups that one surgery inpatient unit held quarterly with previous patients and family members.

Patient/Family Focus Group in Hospital

1. Welcome and purpose: In our effort to provide our patients and their families with a high-quality health care experience, we want to hear what's important to you. We've invited you here today to find out the following:
   —What you liked most and least about your experience with us
   —What you would suggest we change to make it a better hospital
   —Feedback about some particular aspects of your care that we want to know about, so we can make improvements
2. Introductions
3. Ground rules
   —Confidentiality: Ask, "Can we audiotape this, to help us remember everything you said and develop an accurate report? Also, may I take notes?"
   —What we'll do with the results
   —Length

—Food, payment?

—Tell them, "Anything goes; the more candid you are, the more we learn."

4. In your experience with us, what stands out as the high points? What did you appreciate most?

5. In your experience with us, what bothered you? What frustrated you? What was disturbing or annoying or irritating or upsetting?

6. What happened that made you anxious during your experience with us?
   —What steps if any did staff take to ease your anxiety?
   —What else could they have done to ease your anxiety?

7. Some of you might have entered through the emergency room. Some might not. Who did? What was your experience like there?
   —Pluses
   —Minuses

8. Some of you had surgery and some did not. If you had surgery, what was your experience before and after surgery?
   —How would you evaluate the education or preparation process
      –Before surgery (helpful, not helpful, missing)
      –Told about sleeping
      –IVs and other tubes
      –What to expect regarding pain ·
      –Pain/nausea medications and availability?
      –Blood pressure, pulse, heart rate checked?
      –Expected to cough and do deep breathing?
      –Risks and benefits?

9. After surgery, what happened that was helpful, not helpful, missing?
   —Before going home, what happened that was helpful, not helpful, missing?
   —Those of you who went home with dressing changes, tubes, central lines, what were you educated about? What was overlooked? What questions did you have later?
   —What would you have liked to know about resuming activities?
   —Was time spent educating your family? On what? What was missing?

10. What were your experiences here for services or treatments other than surgery?
    —Evaluate the education or preparation you received
       –Before treatment (helpful, unhelpful, missing pieces)
       –About risks and benefits

–During your treatment

–After treatment

In preparation for going home, what would you have liked to know about resuming activities? What would have helped?

11. To what extent do you think people went out of their way for you? Examples?
12. Missed opportunities?
13. Handling of delays:
    —When did you experience them?
    —Which were most bothersome?
    —Were you given reasons?
    —Do you recall the reasons for delays?
14. Give us a grade in our behavior toward your family/friends and explain.
15. Physical comforts?
16. Admissions process?
17. If you ran this hospital, how would you change it?
18. Anything else you want to tell us?
19. Closing
    —What we'll do with what we learned from you . . .
    —Gratitude for their willingness to come and talk openly about their experience.

For a medical practice try this:

1. Introductions; your experience with our practice: number of years, who in your family, how you heard about it initially.
2. Think back to the last time you had some kind of interaction with our practice. Could we go around and have people say a bit about the situation and how you felt about it?
3. In your experiences with our practice, what have you liked?
4. In your experience with our practice, what haven't you liked?
5. Can you think of specific situations that you wish the doctor had handled differently?
6. How do you feel about the office environment? What could we do to improve it?
7. How do you feel about office systems, like scheduling appointments, phone, billing, and so on? How could we improve these?

8. How would you rate this practice on the following:
—Amenities or extras provided to make you feel comfortable
—Personal attention and responsiveness to you
—Staff courtesy
—Physician attention
—Convenience
—Access to the doctor when you want it
—The way people handle billing/money situations
9. If you owned this practice, how would you improve it?

6. Do the groundwork to get people there.
7. Identify staff and prepare them to attend.
—Draw straws, invite volunteers, or use some appropriate criteria to identify which staff members should attend to listen. Arrange for their attendance.
—Hold a prep session for them in which you make clear their role as listeners, not participants (until the end when the facilitator will ask them if they have any follow-up questions for the customer group).
—Also, coach them to take notes, with instructions to write down everything they hear, not their interpretations of what they hear. Emphasize that they'll meet later to revisit and share what they heard and to summarize and draw conclusions from it.
8. During the session, remind staff to take copious notes of what they hear (not what they interpret about what they hear). Facilitator tips:
—Throughout, the facilitator needs to use reflective listening and paraphrasing to make sure people are clear about what is being said.
—After one person answers, the facilitator should invite other responses with cues like, "How do other people see this?" or "To what extent do people agree with that?" or "Does anyone see this differently?"
—He or she should use positive, accepting nonverbal behavior, saying "Uh-huh," "Yes?" and nodding to encourage people to express themselves.
—And he or she should probe and push but at no time disagree with what someone says.

9. Convene those staff who attended in a follow-up meeting within a week of the group. Ask people to bring their notes. In the meeting, ask people questions that help them share what they heard, and *afterward* draw conclusions about it. List each question on a flipchart and record responses.
   —For each question ask, "What did you hear?" and record
   –Customer feelings
   –Customer thoughts
   –Customer suggestions
   —Note the patterns that emerge and ask the following questions:
   –"Looking at these, how do you feel in response?"
   –"What do you consider the central issues in what you heard? What's at the heart of what you heard?"
   –"What conclusions do you draw?"
   –"What are the implications for our service? Where might this lead us? What might we start doing, continue doing, stop doing, or improve/change?"

10. Ask staff who attended to prepare their results to make a presentation to the rest of their team who did not attend the group. Ask staff also to facilitate a discussion among their team about what impressed them, disturbed them, enlightened them, and what ideas they have about what to do with what they learned.

11. Have staff give the presentation, listen to their colleagues, and make plans for follow-up.

12. Convene the staff who attended and process and evaluate the whole experience.
    —What did they think and feel when listening to their customers?
    —What about the process helped them listen and learn?
    —What stood in the way?
    —What did they learn about themselves in the process?
    —What suggestions do they have for greater effectiveness with the next wave of customer focus groups?

 Tips

- Rotate staff participation so, over time, many people get a chance to attend. Jump through whatever hoops necessary to enable staff to go, for example, giving them released work time, paying them overtime—whatever it takes because your service and customers will benefit greatly.

- Consider a system of regular focus groups, for instance, one group per month or one group per quarter.
- Consider also a focus group for *each* customer group. Do another with referral sources. Do one with group purchasers of your services, such as payers or employer groups.
- Don't fall into the trap of thinking that you already know what customers think. Focus groups that produce nothing eye-opening are, to say the least, few and far between. If you hold a focus group and learn nothing, you need to make sure that your questions are open ended and clear, and that you are prepared to probe for depth, for thoughts and feelings, and go beyond people's first response.
- A schedule of periodic focus groups is better than one focus group session. It's easy to forget to get feedback. That's why you need to build feedback gathering into your service on a systematic, regular, nonhaphazard basis—monthly, weekly, quarterly. Then, you don't forget.
- Don't worry about using methods that are research-pure or unobtrusive. The methods described here have proven effective in evoking valuable, usable, face-valid information. Also, when you are blatant about what you're trying to learn, you not only gather usable information; you also communicate to your respondents that you care what they think and are dedicated to making your service meet their needs—even to the point of inviting negative comments. Regarding obtrusiveness, the more you and your staff ask for patient satisfaction feedback, the more your minds will be focused on taking all possible steps to achieve patient satisfaction. The questions implant in your mind a service orientation that tends to attune you to patients and their needs. It's all to the better if the existence of these questions makes you more responsive to patients before you get a chance to measure their perceptions. The goal is to optimize satisfaction in every way.

A Promise

You will be amazed at what focus groups like these do for your team. Staff hear about their own impact from the horse's mouth.

Then, being good people, they will let customer voices echo in their minds and influence how they go about their daily work.

These methods help frontline staff hear the voice of the customer directly. That's the ideal, since few staff members dispute what they hear when they hear it firsthand. Because most staff members have very positive intentions about helping others and meeting their patients' and other customers' needs, when they hear feedback first-hand, they tend to consciously or unconsciously respond to it by making course corrections.

Adopting the Customer's Perspective in Everyday Work

Another set of tools that helps people hear and use the customer's voice as a guide doesn't engage staff in consulting customers. These tools engage staff in taking on or adopting a customer point of view. They help staff look at services through the lens of a customer. They encourage the use of role-playing and empathy.

Here are three such tools:

- Saint Francis Care's "Through Our Patients' Eyes" program
- Staff as mystery shoppers
- Simulated customer experiences

 ### Saint Francis Care's "Through Our Patients' Eyes" Program

This tool provides all managers with a close, personal understanding of the customer experience by placing them in the position of customer and also observer in patient-customer interactions. It was adapted from a wonderful program that Saint Francis Hospital and Medical Center in Hartford, Connecticut, developed for its Saint Francis Care managers. Every manager was asked to select and complete three exercises from among these two types:

1. *Service area exercises:* In these exercises, each manager observes one employee throughout a variety of patient-customer inter-actions. For instance, the manager observes an employee who provides the reception function, the billing function, or a clean-ing function.Or they observe many patients experiencing the same step in a service cycle, such as reception, a blood draw, or an explanation of discharge instructions.

Service Area Exercise Example

Service Area Name: Admission/Registration
Service Area Liaison: Liz Cunha, x45664
Service Area Location: 2d floor, PCT

Exercise Description: Observe the admission process in the admissions office. See the interaction of admission staff with patients and their families regarding registration information, insurance, and so on. A key component is to assimilate information about the patients' concerns and anxieties as they enter the hospital.

Exercise duration: Two hours
Special restrictions: None

Reprinted, with permission, from Saint Francis Hospital & Medical Center, Hartford, CT, © 1997

2. *Patient episode exercises:* In these exercises, the manager follows a single patient (with the patient's permission) through a series of interactions with the service over time, related to a single episode of care. For instance, the manager might observe one cardiac patient's experience during the admission process, before and after surgery, and during the discharge process.

Patient Episode Exercise Example

Area Name: Cardiology
Liaison: Steve Rosen, x44060

Exercise Description: Observe the process of a patient undergoing an elective outpatient cardiac catheter. Observe the admission process from admitting to the cardiac unit. Observe the process of admitting the patient to the floor, preparation for cardiac catheter, and the procedure. Follow the patient back to cardiac unit for recovery and discharge.

Note: During this exercise, you should accompany the patient during the discharge process. It is your responsibility to communicate with appropriate staff and to accompany the patient during discharge.

Exercise: Open ended (total process six to eight hours)
Specific Restrictions: none

Reprinted, with permission, from Saint Francis Hospital & Medical Center, Hartford, CT, © 1997

Another patient episode exercise asks the observer to follow an MRI patient from start to finish and also experience the procedure personally as part of the experience. The manager shadows the patient or employee and observes. Afterward, within 24 hours, the manager is required to participate in a debriefing session (at least 20 minutes long) with the service area liaison and staff host, during which they discuss the experience and brainstorm recommendations. Then, within 10 days, the manager completes a management team member documentation form about the area observed, which includes

- Key observations/findings
- Improvement opportunities
- Recommendations

These forms are compiled, reviewed, and ultimately distributed to all department or service heads.

Method
You can adapt this approach to your organization whether it is large like a hospital/network or at least big enough to have people in various positions performing their functions where others on the team aren't characteristically able to watch.

1. Select an orchestrator of the program—someone with a strong stake in customer service improvement and a position of credibility in relation to your organization's managers (for example, an educator, marketing professional, organization development professional, human resources professional, or administrator). This person, acting as developer/facilitator, convenes all managers and provides an overview of the program.
2. Conduct an overview of the approach for all managers.
3. Have managers related to different services develop exercises that other managers can complete in their area, including guidelines for interacting with patients appropriately during the exercise. Gather these in a booklet for all to read in preparation for requesting their preferred assignments.
4. Circulate the booklet to all managers, and invite people to fill out a form that tells their first, second, and third choices of exercises in areas in which they are least familiar already.

5. Have the facilitator match managers to their preferred exercises and provide a time frame. The facilitator then provides each manager with background information about the service that they will be observing.

6. Staff liaisons proceed to contact managers to schedule their exercises.

7. Managers do their exercises, completing a feedback report afterward for the liaison and host in the area observed and also providing a written report for later distribution to all managers.

Variation

Although this program works best in an organization large enough to have various departments or services run by different managers, if your service is not large enough to have various work teams and managers, adapt this approach to frontline staff in your service. Ask staff members in different positions to develop the exercises and have every staff member do an exercise in relation to a part of your service least familiar to them.

Tips

- This is a very powerful way to help managers and staff adopt a customer perspective—as they observe someone else's service. By focusing on someone else's service, they are less defensive and more observant than they would be about their own service. Yet, the happy fact is that the experience helps them, at the same time, develop perspective on their own service.

- Engage staff and teams in developing the exercises. That's the only way to make the exercises realistic, rich, and doable. People close to the service need to define the parameters.

Staff as Mystery Shoppers

The mystery shopper approach also employs staff or other friends of your service as observers and consultants. You've undoubtedly heard of the mystery shopper programs used to evaluate retail stores, restaurants, airlines, hotels, and the like. The key concept is that people experience the service, and unbeknownst to the service providers, they observe certain quality features.

You can build a simple program of this type that provides your service with feedback from people in a planned, purposeful way when your staff doesn't know anyone is experiencing their services with a critical eye.

Method

Involve your staff in *all* of the following decisions:

1. Identify those aspects of your service that a person using the service can evaluate.
2. Decide which of these aspects are conducive to a mystery shopper approach (those that someone can experience in a short period of time without engaging in invasive procedures or risk).
3. Develop a tool that structures the observer's observations, such as the following:

Mystery Shopper Phone Call

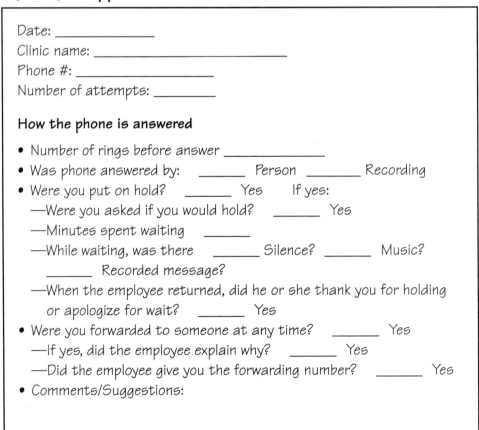

Date: _____

Clinic name: _____

Phone #: _____

Number of attempts: _____

How the phone is answered

- Number of rings before answer _____
- Was phone answered by: _____ Person _____ Recording
- Were you put on hold? _____ Yes If yes:
  —Were you asked if you would hold? _____ Yes
  —Minutes spent waiting _____
  —While waiting, was there _____ Silence? _____ Music?
  _____ Recorded message?
  —When the employee returned, did he or she thank you for holding or apologize for wait? _____ Yes
- Were you forwarded to someone at any time? _____ Yes
  —If yes, did the employee explain why? _____ Yes
  —Did the employee give you the forwarding number? _____ Yes
- Comments/Suggestions:

Greeting

- Did the employee say his or her name? If yes, who was it?

  _____

- Greeting used: _____
- Did the employee have a pleasant tone? _____ Yes
- Did the employee offer help? _____ Yes
- Were you asked for your name? _____ Yes
- Was your name used by employee? _____ Yes
  If yes, how often? _____
- If you called for an appointment, did the employee ask the following:
  —About insurance? _____ Yes
  —If this was first visit? _____ Yes
  —How you were referred? _____ Yes
  —The purpose of the appointment? _____ Yes
  —If you needed directions? _____ Yes
  —Other information? _____
- Comments/Suggestions:

End of Call

- Were you thanked for calling? _____ Yes
- Did the employee say good-bye? _____ Yes
- Were you left with a good feeling? _____ Yes
- Good-bye comment_____
- Comments/Suggestions:

Overall

- Was the speaker
  —Courteous? _____ Yes
  —Professional? _____ Yes
  —Attentive? _____ Yes
  —Helpful? _____ Yes
- How satisfied were you with the handling of the call?
  _____ Very Satisfied _____ Somewhat Satisfied
  _____ Neutral _____ Not Very Satisfied
  _____ Not at all Satisfied
- Comments/Suggestions:

4. Identify people who might serve as mystery shoppers, such as volunteers, staff from another service, or consumers from a group with a stake in the effectiveness of your service. Ask them if they will serve as mystery shoppers for you. Specify the time required and the nature of the task.

5. Identify staff who will process the forms and provide results to the team quickly, with an opportunity to discuss the significance and possible follow-up actions.

6. In order to avoid generating distrust and fear in the organization, communicate with everyone in the organization that a mystery shopper program is going to start. Explain its importance to service improvement. Tell people you don't want to do it without them knowing that it's happening.

7. Set up and provide training for the people who will serve as mystery shoppers.

8. Set up a feedback loop to staff and determine your plan for using the feedback to trigger improvements.

9. Set up a baseline for measuring your service's success. Develop markers for improvement and plot these on a 6- to 12-month chart that shows your mystery shoppers' findings. This will give staff improvement goals and enable you to track progress together.

 Tips

- The fact is, when staff are involved in designing the mystery shopper program, they learn what is being evaluated, and this might cause them to improve their behavior immediately. Great! Let them all know what's being tested, since your goal is impressive service, not catching people behaving badly.

- Keep the observation forms detailed so you learn more than you know. And allow for comments and suggestions from the observer.

 ### Simulated Customer Experiences

Simulated customer experiences are another approach to introducing the customer's voice into your service. You can create experiences within a classroom environment to give staff a firsthand experience of being a patient. These experiences build empathy for patient feelings and concerns. Two activities you can use to develop customer simulations with your staff are experience skits and blindfold exercises.

Activity: Experience Skits

In staff meetings or special sessions, experience skits can help staff adopt a customer perspective on rough spots in your service.

1. With staff, generate a list of specific services or points along the patient's pathway through your services where complaints are common.
2. Select from the list those service points that can be simulated in the classroom.
3. Divide your group into subgroups. Within each subgroup, assign roles so that some people are caregivers and others are the patient, family member, or others on the receiving end of the service cycle.
4. Have these subgroups simultaneously run the patient through the service step.
5. Afterward, invite everyone's feelings and suggestions.
6. Then, as a group, generate ways to improve that step in the service cycle as a result of patient experiences with an eye to reducing complaints about that step.

Consider focusing this process on one service point per staff meeting, so that every meeting provides some practice in adopting the viewpoint of patients or other customers. As you repeat this process, staff get used to it and the process runs itself.

Activity: Blindfold Exercise

Use this tool in a workshop designed to build staff empathy for patients' experiences. Ideally, have someone with group process skills help facilitate this experience. So that you have enough people (at least 10), invite another manager to join you with his or her staff and also help you run the exercise.

1. Supplies needed: Two flipcharts and pads, markers, blindfolds (enough for half the group), tape or CD player, and a CD or tape with soft music.

2. Leader/facilitator gives every other person a blindfold, making sure that there is an even number of people, with half blindfolded and half not. Ask people with blindfolds who are wearing glasses to place them where they will be safe. Have people put on their blindfolds and make sure they can't see. Tell people that they must be silent once their blindfold is on.

3. Ask the blindfolded people to sit quietly and alert them by saying, "[Name the person] is here to make sure you aren't talking, while I talk with the sighted people out in the hallway."

4. When sighted people are outside with you, give these instructions: Each sighted person is supposed to enter the room and take a blindfolded person on a 10-minute walk. At the end of 10 minutes, they are supposed to return and take a different blindfolded person on a walk for 5 minutes. Say, "I'll let you know when 10 minutes are up by ringing a bell, and then I'll ring it again after the next 5 minutes. Each time, bring your person back into the room and sit them down."

5. It's very important to let them know two rules: (1) They cannot talk to the blindfolded person, and (2) they must keep them safe.

6. They may ask the following questions:
   —"If we can't talk, how do we get them to go up and down stairs?" Ask the group for ideas (for example, you can stomp your foot, touch the person's leg, or otherwise show through touch that the person needs to take a step down).
   —"Did you give the blindfolded people any directions?" The answer is no.

7. Don't spend too much time answering more questions. Tell them the directions one more time and send them off. Tell them that if they stay in the vicinity, they'll see you wave when it's time to come back. As they return for the last time, turn on the tape recorder or CD player to soft music until everyone is in the room and you're ready to help them process their experience.

8. Help people talk about and learn from the experience.
   —When everyone is back, ask the blindfolded staff to remove their blindfolds. There will be a lot of laughing and chattering; let it be for a minute or so.
   —Tell them that you would like to have them talk about their experiences. Let them know that you are going to start by asking the blindfolded people first to describe their experience (their thoughts, feelings, and actions), and then

the people who guided them will have a chance to share their experiences.

—Focus on their experience for a while before bringing up any correlation between being a patient and being a blindfolded person. You will hear things like the following: "It was hard for me to understand what was going on. I had a hard time at first, but then I just started trusting the person guiding me and I relaxed. I was really aware of my senses. I had to rely on my other senses more since I couldn't see or talk."

—Once a few people have shared, introduce the patient into the discussion. Say, "Now I would like everyone to think about the experience as if the blindfolded staff were the patient or plan member. Talk about your experience being blindfolded as it relates to patients' experiences in our service. How are patient experiences similar to this? How are they different?" Some of the responses may be like the following: "I can see why patients feel so worried about what we might do, particularly if we don't communicate with them about each detail of what we are doing. I can see why we make up what management is going to do when we may not be told the whole story."

—Feel free to comment and add your own thoughts. Also, dig deeper at opportune times. For instance, if someone shares frustration about not being able to communicate with their guide, push them on how this applies to patients and what they can do about it.

—Give the guides/caregivers a chance to talk about their experiences. They'll talk about the responsibility they felt while guiding the blindfolded person. Dig for discussion about their frustrations and what they can do about them with patients. They might talk about not knowing how to approach the blindfolded person or that they wanted the person to have a great experience but couldn't control it, or that the person didn't seem to trust them. Talk about issues related to control, dependency, choice, respect, and dignity, emphasizing ways caregivers can optimize these for patients.

—Invite people to share what they learned from this activity. Reinforce the importance of taking the patient viewpoint on their work, so that they remember how the patients might feel and respond in their dependent roles. Finally, thank people wholeheartedly for participating.

The following are some tips that can make the blindfold exercise more effective:

- Because this exercise can sensitize staff to the issues they take for granted with patients/families/staff members, encourage them to take the information they learn and use it to make improvements in their communication with customers and thereby affect their satisfaction with your service.
- In future staff meetings, refer to the blindfold experience when talking about a patient's concern or complaint. Make comments like, "This patient felt blindfolded. Remember how that felt?" References to the blindfolding experience will become shorthand for reminding people to adopt their patients' perspectives and feelings.

Maintaining the Customer Perspective

The challenge now is to help staff actually use their refined role-taking skills in their everyday work, not just in the classroom or in specially structured situations. Years ago at a conference, one of the authors, Wendy Leebov, noticed a brass plate in front of a gentleman at the conference table. The brass plate read *bwatp*. This gentleman sat there all day with that plate in front of him, without commenting about it. At the end of the day, Wendy asked, "What does *bwatp* mean?" He answered, "It means 'But what about the patient?'" He explained that most meetings of health care professionals focus on anything *but* the patient—on finances, rules, policies, reimbursement, cost cutting, accreditation visits, reengineering, mergers, and the like. He made himself this brass plate so that he could stop any group meeting in its tracks and, while pointing to the sign, say, "Excuse me. Please read my sign. It says *bwatp* and that stands for 'But what about the patient'! We seem to have forgotten the patient in this discussion." And lo and behold, he said, the discussion would shift. This man used a gimmick creatively to help people remember the patient during their everyday work.

Give some thought with your team to developing your own gimmicks to help the patient remain present in the room when you're making decisions, planning, and solving problems. If the patient could only be there in that room, so many service-related decisions would be better—in the interest of the patient.

Here are two tools that you might adopt as is or use with staff to design your own:

1. Job aid to remember to "Think customer"
2. Mike Ustomer

Job Aid to Remember to "Think Customer"

This tool strikes people as so simple as to be unnecessary. It asks you to think like your customers when you're entertaining some new possibility or solution. But the fact is, the biggest problem when we evaluate options or think of solutions is that we often forget to adopt a customer perspective. We forget to ask, "How will our customers react to this?"

Method

1. Post this job aid in a prominent place in your work area.

Job Aid: Through Our Customers' Eyes

1. Who exactly is impacted by the proposed course of action? Which customers?
   —Patients
   —Their families
   —Caregivers
   —Referrers
   —Payers
   —Internal customers
   —Other customer groups
2. What would each customer group be likely to think and feel about this course of action? How would they evaluate its potential impact? Thinking like them, is there another course of action that they would prefer?

(P.S. If you aren't sure how to answer these questions, don't guess. Consult your customers to find out their thoughts and feelings!)

Reprinted, with permission, from Saint Francis Hospital & Medical Center, Hartford, CT, © 1997

2. Push yourself to read it when you're thinking through ideas, developing proposals, evaluating options, and making decisions.

3. If you can't answer the questions by assuming your customers' perspectives, use a direct method, such as interviews, focus groups, or surveys, to solicit feedback from your customers.

Tips

• Post this on your blotter, your phone, your office door, or your date book. Put it somewhere where it stares you in the face and reminds you of the important customer question. In time, hopefully, you'll see it in your sleep and can throw away the frayed paper on which it's written!

• Carry around extras, perhaps on a business card, and give them to staff or coworkers who you think also need to ask these questions.

Mike Ustomer

This tool is powerful and fun. It adds variety and whimsy to your discussions and work. At the same time, it helps you and your team to allow the customer's voice into your discussions and decision-making processes.

This tool has three purposes:

1. To remind staff of the thoughts, feelings, and needs of their customers when they are making decisions, changes, or improvements.

2. To help staff pinpoint and articulate what they already know about the thoughts, feelings, and needs of their customers

3. To help staff share different perspectives on the thoughts, feelings, and needs of their customers

Method

1. Purchase or find someone to make a large (preferably life-size) floppy doll. The doll should be as plain as possible, so that you can dress it, giving it a variety of characteristics or personalities. Dress the doll to represent a typical customer for your service.

2. Bring the doll to a staff meeting. Introduce this doll as the symbol of a typical customer of your service.

—Say, "We've been actively involved in finding out what our customers need and want from us, and we've learned a great deal from these activities." Point out some of the things the team learned, or ask people to share what they learned.

—Continue, "These insights have helped us refine our plans for improving our systems and our services." Again, draw the relationship to several of the efforts the team made to improve service and their insights into what customers need and want.

—Finally, say, "I know we'll continue to include and involve customers directly for a long time. But there are times when I think we either forget what we already know about what our customers need and want, or we don't use the information at the right time. Usually, this happens when we're together in planning sessions or staff meetings, and, for obvious reasons, we need to do something to correct this."

3. Introduce Mike to the group, telling them that Mike has offered to come to these important group meetings and, when appropriate, share his feelings and ideas.

4. Tell the group that Mike is here at this meeting to give it a try, but that he wants input from the group at the end of the meeting about how he can be most helpful. At this point, your team will probably be somewhat skeptical or giggly, but persist. Go on with your meeting as planned.

5. Whenever group discussions involve sharing ideas and suggestions for change, turn to Mike and ask him to respond to the ideas on the floor. Have people speak for Mike, sharing how the idea or issue would affect him as a customer. Ask a staff member to pretend to be Mike and answer the questions as she or he believes Mike would.

6. If people become stymied about a question or decision, ask the group if anyone can suggest what Mike might advise. If no one can comfortably speak as Mike, ask the group how they can get from their real customers the information or opinions they're unable to guess.

7. At the end of the meeting, ask the group to evaluate the use of Mike as a way to remember their customers' voices. Discuss ways to use Mike's presence better in future meetings.

Variations

- Figure out with your team simple ways to change the doll to represent each of several of your customer groups. Then, ask your team at each meeting which customer group the doll should represent because of the nature of the meeting.
- Another twist on this activity is having doll customers participate in small group activities. It might be too expensive to purchase and equip multiple dolls, but you can use balloons for small group work. Give each small group a balloon. Tell them that this balloon is a customer. As their first task, ask them to give this customer a name and a profile or point of view. Also, provide markers so people can put a face on their balloon. As the meeting continues, ask individuals in each group to take turns holding the balloons. When holding the balloon, the staff member speaks as the customer.

Tips

- Remember, the purpose of this activity is to include the voice of the customer in our daily work. The idea is to teach staff how to use the information about their customers that they already have and to remember that they need to consult customers when they don't have a very good reason to think they can speak for them.
- People will respond well to this technique if you present it well. You might need to resolve any feelings you have that this is silly, contrived, or gimmicky. If you feel that way, your staff will know it and also become uncomfortable.
- Engage your team in dressing up the doll and naming it, so that they feel connected to it.
- Using a doll works very well in strategic and future planning sessions. It won't be as important for simple, small group-sharing sessions. Encourage people to give Mike a name and personality that more closely match their customers'.
- Again, every time you try a new approach with your team, ask, "In what ways was this helpful and not helpful? And how can we improve it?"
- Props that remind your team of their customers' presence don't have to be time consuming, expensive, or clever. They just have to help staff adopt the mind-set of their customers.

Conclusion

If only we used the discipline to see our services through our customers' eyes, not through our eyes as providers, we would almost automatically make improvements in these services, and in the process have a dramatic impact on customer satisfaction. Some people are gifted when it comes to role taking. Others are not. If you want your staff to make significant improvements in service, be their fitness coach and help them build role-taking muscles, muscles they flex in order to see the world through their customers' eyes.

Chapter 4

• • •

Remove Barriers so Staff Can Serve Customers

Do You Need to Read This Chapter?

Read these case studies and see if any sound familiar. If you face situations like these, you'll definitely benefit from reading on.

- Tony the technician spent his own money to purchase T-shirts for his group during Radiology Week. He wanted to show his appreciation to coworkers for working so hard on the redesign effort. He knew everyone was under a great deal of pressure and the team needed a boost. When he brought in the shirts, his boss told him that although it was a nice gesture, the hospital dress code prohibited wearing T-shirts, and he should have asked permission beforehand.

- One day, Mary, a receptionist in a group practice, faced a dilemma when a physician left early because of a family emergency. The other doctors were completely booked, so she called all of this doctor's patients to see if they would be willing to reschedule. Except for two patients who had already left for their appointments, she was successful. When she reported her success to the office manager, she was reprimanded for not discussing it with the manager and the other physicians before she made the calls. Mary tried to explain that she knew most of the patients and she was concerned about meeting their needs and avoiding inconveniencing them, but her supervisor said, "We are running a business here, and the goal is to see as many patients as possible. You shouldn't have canceled anyone."

- Nancy, an office manager, was very upset the day an angry customer blew into the office and carried on in the waiting area about a billing problem. Nancy first tried to calm the customer down, then to move him to a more private location, but he was adamant and loud about speaking to her boss immediately. Unfortunately, her boss was out of the office at a meeting and wouldn't return for an hour. Not only was the customer determined to wait; he was determined to make the office staff miserable in the meantime. Nancy didn't know what she could do to solve the problem.

- Karen, a new manager, is trying to grasp how her team works. From the start, her staff complained of being overworked and short-staffed. The way Karen sees it, the group is used to working in an environment with poor work processes that make efficiency impossible. People spend a great deal of time looking for supplies, looking for lost items, retrieving borrowed equipment, and taking things from each other's areas. Unfortunately, the group seems unwilling to address the issue, claiming, "It's just the way things are around here," and "We can't do anything about it."

- Susan, a nurse, often feels caught between helping patients and following policies and procedures. When she tries to bring this up at staff meetings, she gets cut off and shut down. She can't even get anyone to help her understand why a particular policy has been created. The history seems to be "Don't ask, just do."

- Frank, who works in maintenance, has had it with his coworkers. He thinks they're pigs who never clean up after themselves and have no respect for the team or their environment. The place is such a mess that no one can find anything they need. It's become so bad that he now feels he has to lock up his own equipment to protect it.

Do any of these scenarios sound familiar? Unfortunately, these stories and more are the norm in many health care organizations. And who loses? Everyone. Staff are frustrated because they feel that the system, their bosses, their coworkers, and even the environment get in the way of meeting their customers' needs. Customers see the systems and procedures as designed for the convenience of the provider, not for them. And bosses feel overwhelmed with what to do about these barriers. Often, they don't know where to begin.

It's Confusing!

The question is how to free up staff to meet the needs of their customers. There are so many barriers. You need to make sure that the environment is designed and managed in a way that staff have ready access to the tools they need when serving customers. You must decide how you want staff to spend their time and energy, making sure that they don't have to jump through hoops or get stuck in red tape to do it, all the while respecting that nothing and no one is perfect, and that staff need to know what they can do and who they can turn to when inevitable glitches occur. And even if you make improvements by removing barriers that block staff efforts to serve their customers, changes have a mysterious way of reverting to their original chaotic state.

How to Remove Barriers

First of all, you must get your team's attention. That's not easy because many people, although they don't tend to admit it, find comfort in the status quo. Despite the frustrations caused by barriers to serving customers, there are also benefits from these barriers that make them very tough to change.

What are the benefits for staff of keeping the barriers to service delivery in place? Consider the following chart:

Staff Description of a Barrier to Service Delivery	Benefits of Keeping the Barrier in Place
This place is a mess.	• I don't need to clean up after myself. • If I can't find something, I have something or someone else to blame. • I always have a ready excuse for why I can't get my work done. • I don't have to go to the trouble of replenishing supplies, reporting a shortage, or keeping to a system because no one else does.

These policies don't make any sense!	• I don't tend to think for myself because here it is in black and white. • If a customer complains about the way we do things, I have a ready reply. I can point to the policy. • I don't need to worry about how others interpret a problem or situation because they have the answer in front of them.
I'm never sure what they want me to do and not do around here!	• I don't need to think for myself. I just let the higher-ups worry about it. • I don't need to get involved in sticky situations. I'll just let someone else worry about it. • If I don't act, I won't stand the chance of getting in trouble. • I can blame confusion about what I'm allowed to do for not going out of my way to do anything.

The point is, in subtle and not-so-subtle ways, some managers and staff benefit from perpetuating systems' problems, inconveniences, unclear guidelines, and other barriers to efficient, proactive service delivery. These barriers are very hard nuts to crack.

Start with You

The first nut you might need to crack concerns your own motives and bias against action. If you are determined to remove barriers for staff, it's going to take work, for all of you. It's difficult to help people see their part in perpetuating the barriers, and developing new systems and work processes is time consuming. It will take time to clarify guidelines for action and to keep any changes in place.

Are you determined to remove barriers to your staff's serving their customers? Let's look at the potential benefits.

• If you work with staff to create systems that remove inconveniences (like supply shortages), staff will have more time to serve more customers and satisfy them better. And you'll have more time to focus on the more important aspects of your job, such as future planning, developing your staff, and cultivating new business and relationships, rather than putting out fires and handling routine, repeated customer complaints.

- If you clarify guidelines for what staff can and cannot do without approval and loosen up those guidelines, staff will learn to rely more on each other for solving problems, will hound you less, and will develop better internal customer relationships.
- If you remove barriers, staff can focus on developing better customer relations skills. They'll feel better about their abilities to handle problems independently, and they won't have excuses as to why they can't serve their customers well.
- If you make it easier for staff to serve their customers, there will be fewer problems with customers. You'll have improved or removed the conditions that create hassles in the first place.

Finally, and most important, customers are going to be happier with you and your service, and they will spread the good word about your people and your service. And that means a more loyal customer following, which is critical in today's market.

What to Do?

If only there were magic wands, potions, or recipes for removing barriers to effective, efficient service delivery. Although there aren't panaceas, a lot of small initiatives can cumulatively remove significant barriers. The following strategies will chip away at the barriers to service delivery:

- Create a more user-friendly environment with and for staff.
- Rethink your policies and procedures so they don't stop staff from doing right by customers.
- Clarify boundaries to help staff discover and refine what they can and can't do in typical, everyday situations to meet customer needs.
- Tackle other barriers that staff can identify.
- Develop backup plans staff can use when service breaks down.

The following sections discuss each of these strategies in detail, and offer concrete tools and tips for accomplishing them.

Create a More User-Friendly Environment with and for Staff

Think about how difficult it is to accommodate customers if you're missing supplies, equipment, forms, or other necessary items. Do your staff enter their work spaces and clear them up, so that they can start working? Is everything they need in place and easy to find, or do they spend loads of time looking for something or moving piles of work from place to place? Do people leave equipment broken without reporting it or arranging for a replacement? Does your team feel good about their physical environment?

Staff need to feel their space is in order and that they can find the tools they need to serve their customers. Typically, several people share a work space, so they need to agree about how to organize the space so that it serves everyone, and they need to commit to maintaining whatever systems are set up.

Staff not only want functional places to do their work, they want them to look and feel good. Are there appealing aspects to the environment, like flowers, music (if appropriate), an absence of clutter?

What a difference it can make to your internal and your external customers if staff are ready to go to work the moment they come into their work area! Make a difference in their workplace by asking their help in removing barriers to services that have to do with their work space and the tools they need.

Work Space Fix

Help your team rethink their work space and make changes for two reasons:

1. So that everyone knows where to find supplies
2. So that staff members *trust* that these supplies will be there when they look for them

This will free up staff to serve customers, instead of spending time frantically looking for equipment, forms, and supplies.

Method

1. Bring staff together and brainstorm a list of their most frustrating moments when trying to find things, such as forms, equipment, or supplies. Give examples to show that anything goes, as in the following:

Frustrations When Trying to Find Things

Which of these are true for this team?

- Is the stapler out of staples when you go to use it?
- Was the last form taken from the shelf and now the shelf is empty—and you have to go search for the original or a fresh supply in a back room?
- When you try to take a phone message, do you find that a colleague walked off with your pen or borrowed it for a minute and didn't return it?
- Do you return to your work area and find someone lolling in your chair?
- Is the computer down, so you can't do your work?
- Did someone forget to replenish the supply closet, so there are no tablets when you need a new one?
- Did your document fail to print, because the last person who removed their print output left the paper tray empty?
- Do you go to make a copy and find that the last person left the machine with an unfixed paper jam?
- Did someone take the patient linen or personal care kits meant for your patients?

Now make a list of your frust rations with your work space.

2. Take this list and create categories, for example, supplies, forms, equipment, clutter, and so on. Place items from the list under the relevant category.
3. Divide the whole group into smaller groups that each take one category and the list of items.
4. Have groups talk about each of the items in the category to figure out the following:

—What can be done to change this?

—How can we tackle the problems?

—What makes sense as three priorities because they are both important and achievable?

5. Reconvene the whole group and ask each small group to report their top three priorities and proposals.

6. Have the group pick priorities for the team that they will commit to accomplishing. Use a multivoting process, where everyone takes a pen and, reviewing the recommendations of all of the small groups, writes down the top three priorities for the team. Read each proposal and ask how many used one of their votes to vote for it. In other words, tally the results right then, so everyone sees the results.

7. With the group's help, figure out how to follow through on the top three priorities. For instance, ask three people to volunteer to chair a miniteam on each priority and develop a plan of action and then bring back their recommendations to the larger group. Or ask people to divide into implementation teams and run with the ball from there.

Here's a sample plan of action:

Problem: Form Management

We never know when the last form has been taken, so we spend all our time looking for a form, while the customer waits and gets annoyed.

Elements to consider:

- Who uses this form?
- Is it just one form that we're talking about, or is it a bigger problem?
- Does everyone know where the forms are kept?
- Is trying to find these forms a problem for everyone who uses them?
- How much time is spent looking for the form?
- Is there no system for how the forms are supposed to stay available?
- If there is a system (in theory), what is it and where does the system break down?

Possible solutions:

• Appoint a monitor every quarter to be responsible for checking on the supply of forms and replenishing it.
• Place a piece of colored paper with the form's name on it at the point in the pile of forms where there are only 25 forms left. When someone takes the form next to the colored paper, they take it and stick it in the mailbox of the quarterly monitor to reorder or replenish the forms. If by some chance, the supply of forms runs out completely, the monitor is also responsible for telling the team when a supply of forms is low and that they need to use another alternative, instead of hunting for forms to no avail.

Tips

• Acknowledge to the team that there are always at least two aspects to problems with the work space. One has to do with the system or method of organization. The other has to do with the people and the degree to which they use or follow that system or method of organization. Encourage staff to address both aspects. It won't help to design great systems with which people don't comply. Encourage your team to make explicit agreements with one another about complying with whatever systems they decide to set up or improve.

• These options help you help staff remove frustrations in their work environment. Now, take action to eliminate barriers created by inappropriate uses of your service's policies and procedures.

Rethink Policies and Procedures so They Don't Stop Staff from Doing Right by Customers

Another barrier that stops staff from serving their customers well concerns rules, policies, and procedures. Does your team tell customers, "I can't. It's against our policy," or "We have a rule against this."

There are two kinds of rules: red rules and green rules. Red rules are rules that cannot be changed. They are either laws, acts of nature, or physically impossible. Green rules are policies, procedures, guidelines, and protocols, and it is possible to change these because they are not laws, they are not acts of nature, and they are not physically impossible.

Customers know the difference. They know we can change green rules if we want to, and they expect us to do so to meet their needs. But, more often than not, frontline service workers go the other way. If they aren't sure whether a rule is red or green, they assume it is red. They play it safe. They protect themselves.

So, while customers expect service workers to ease up on green rules for their sake, many of our employees are busy insisting that these green rules are really red, and using that as a reason why they must say no to the customer. The fact is, ironically, many, many employees have more flexibility than they realize.

Prevent employees from turning green rules into red rules and instead encourage them to ease up on the green rules to satisfy customers *if* they can do so without hurting the organization or other customers.

To remove rules as an overused barrier to meeting customer needs, take time with staff to clarify how and when to enforce and abandon rules to both better serve customer needs and to protect the interests of the organization.

Is This Rule Green or Red?

This tool will help staff distinguish between red and green rules and better understand when they can bend rules or violate policies and guidelines to meet customer needs. It should also reduce CYA (cover-your-assignment) thinking and risk avoidance, which interfere with meeting customer needs.

Method

Hold a staff meeting in which you help staff distinguish between red and green rules and identify situations in which they can bend green rules to satisfy customers.

1. Introduce the concept of green and red rules.
2. Invite staff to think of examples of red rules (for example, No firearms in hospital; no giving of prescription drugs to patient unless licensed to do so) and green rules (No visitors after 9 P.M.; no children in the exam room with a parent).

3. Divide people into pairs. Have pairs interview each other on these questions:

—Which of our rules have you found yourself explaining to customers?

—Which of our rules do you think annoy our customers?

—Which of our rules has prevented you from resolving a customer complaint?

4. Have people share their results. Managers should write each rule on a large Post-It note and stick it to a wall or whiteboard.

5. The manager should create two columns on the board: red rules and green rules.

6. Select one rule at a time, read it, and ask staff which column it goes in. Invite discussion until there is agreement about whether the rule is red or green.

7. Reinforce this point: We are here to satisfy customers whenever we possibly can. While some customers might be upset with some of our red rules, these rules cannot be changed. They are laws, physically impossible for us to change, or acts of nature. But we *can* change green rules, and customers know it. I don't want you to turn green rules into red ones just to play it safe or make it easy for yourself. This infuriates customers, because they *know* the green rules are changeable even when we insist that they are not. So, I want you to really think before you let green rules stop you from satisfying your customers. It's OK to bend green rules if bending them is good for the customer and if it will not create significant problems for the organization or other customers. I realize that making these decisions sounds risky, so, let's talk through some situations to see if we can become more comfortable with bending rules when there's very good reason for the customer's sake.

8. Focus the group on one green rule at a time and ask, "In what circumstances would you think it's appropriate to change this?" Invite examples and comment. Make it clear which rules can be changed if the staff member has very good reasons for the customer's sake without an undue cost or consequence to the organization or other customers. Invite and address questions.

9. Reinforce how important it is to help each other get better at preventing rules from interfering with your initiatives to satisfy customers. Describe future opportunities to discuss case situations where people wondered if they could bend the rules.

Tips

- Push staff to inventory all the rules they tend to discuss with customers. Explore whether they are red or green rules.
- This activity can produce breakthroughs; staff commonly use rules as the excuses for why they can't accommodate customers. Although the discussions can be tedious, stick with them and try to resolve the "yes, buts."
- Ask yourself whether you have a tendency to resort to rules because of a need for control. If so, catastrophize. Imagine the worst-case scenarios and results of relinquishing control to staff. What is the probability that this worst-case scenario would ever happen? Try to create a condition that will protect customers and the team from the worst possibilities, so you can relinquish more control, authority, and decision making to staff. That's the only way they'll feel free to take initiative to satisfy customers.

Clarify Boundaries to Help Staff Discover and Refine What They Can and Can't Do to Meet Customer Needs

To help staff make appropriate judgments about policies and procedures, they need decision-making skills. They need to know what they can and can't do without permission or guidance from you. The lack of clarity around this issue is probably the most difficult, stubborn, and important barrier to the staff's providing better service to customers.

Why is it so difficult to clarify the latitude staff have to make decisions related to meeting customer needs? Think first about why *you* have difficulty (if you do) being completely clear about what you do and don't want staff to do. What's tough for you?

Do you think any of the following?

- You can't spell out every behavior needed or predict every situation to which staff need to respond effectively. So, why bother?
- People and their abilities aren't the same. There are clearly some people whom you know you could trust with just a few guidelines. On the other hand, there are probably employees whom

you couldn't trust to think on their feet, and you feel safer having them come to you with difficult situations, because who knows what they might do.

- You are ultimately responsible. You might feel comfortable letting your people take risks, but you are concerned about your boss. He or she isn't the most supportive administrator when it comes to learning from mistakes.

All these points have elements of truth to them. But if you avoid clarifying what staff can and cannot do and refuse to widen their realm of authority in the process, customers and staff lose out because staff don't take important initiatives to better satisfy customers.

Think as a customer for a minute. Customers want to know that they are in good hands. They want to know that the person serving them can go the distance with them and handle problems that arise. Customers don't like to hear, "I'm not sure; let me ask my supervisor." And, thinking as a customer, you know that once a staff member says this, you think differently (and less) about the staff member. You lose some confidence in them. You might even think, "Why am I dealing with this person? Why don't I just deal with the supervisor?"

On the other hand, think about how impressed you are as a customer when a staff person goes the extra mile, solves a problem, or shows initiative without having to check with anyone.

The following tools will help staff get a better sense of their latitude to act for their customers' sake and will specifically help them develop skills needed to handle sticky situations with customers. The result is that you can trust them more.

 ## Six Degrees of Delegation

This tool will help staff feel comfortable acting independently on behalf of customers.

Method

1. Divide group into smaller groups of three or four.
2. Post "Six Degrees of Delegation" around the room, one per flipchart.

Six Degrees of Delegation

1. Go for it. No need to contact me.
2. Go for it. Tell me what you did.
3. Get permission first. Then, if possible, go for it.
4. Look into the problem. Together, we'll decide what to do.
5. Look into the problem. I'll get more input or approval before deciding what to do.
6. Forget it. This is not something any of us can get involved in right now.

Reprinted, with permissions, from Gail Scott and Associates © 1996

3. Ask teams to walk around the room and on each sheet list examples under two columns: "Appropriate" and "Not Appropriate."
4. Discuss both typical situations and confusing or frustrating situations. Ask what can be done to help people feel more comfortable solving problems.

 Tips

- Don't do this with your staff until you have resolved your own mixed feelings. You certainly don't want to come across as anything but confident—about them and in their ability to be successful.
- Be prepared to share lots of examples. Our experience is that in the beginning, people may only think about the obvious tasks and not search for the opportunities.
- Be sensitive to staff's mixed feelings. They might want some autonomy, but not the responsibility that goes along with it.
- Seek to reach the individuals on your team. Hear them out during this activity. Your team is made up of individuals, so you can't generalize about all of them. Individuals are in different places. Not only do they have different skills and comfort levels, but they also have very different perceptions about what they can and cannot do. You might not be able to figure out six degrees that meet everyone's need. Accept the fact that the discussion you're starting here will have to be ongoing, as will staff understanding about the latitude in their choices.

Sticky Situations

This tool has several purposes:

- To learn from mistakes and problems as a group
- To emphasize the contributions the team can make to every individual's ability to handle sticky service challenges
- To identify tough situations and equip staff with alternative ways to approach them
- To bury the past and move on

Method

1. During monthly staff meetings, reserve a portion of the meeting for solving and discussing sticky situations.
2. Ask individuals or small groups to think of a time during the past month when they were caught between a rock and a hard place or when they weren't sure what to do for their customer.
3. Each small group writes down cases and passes them to another group.
4. The new group discusses the cases and generates possible ways to handle or solve the problems.
5. Groups read their sticky cases to the large group and share their solutions and suggestions.

Variation

Another way to facilitate this process is to ask people during the week or month to think of sticky situations that they feel would be good to discuss as learning opportunities. At the staff meeting ask people to share their stories, what they did at the time, and how they felt about the outcome. These stories can serve several purposes: They can help people learn what others have done in tough situations, thus helping other people to feel comfortable; they can also be a form of Monday morning quarterbacking, or "Now that we are not caught up in the moment, what could have been done?" Consider starting the process by writing sticky situations on Post-It notes beforehand and then, in the session, asking people to pull them out of a hat and take a crack at solutions. You can, of course, include situations you think are sticky and good learning opportunities.

Tips

- Obviously, the point is to learn, and you have to be very clear about the ground rules.
- This is not about blaming and finger pointing. Stop it immediately if you see any of that behavior. If you don't stop it, the group will distrust the process and shut down permanently.

Tackle Other Barriers That Staff Can Identify

Unanticipated barriers often emerge, and you can't plan for everything. That's why the next tools are versatile for identifying and tackling other barriers that don't fall within any of the above categories. Consider holding potluck staff meetings in which you cast a wide net and invite staff to identify whatever problems they think impede service and to develop solutions. Here's your chance to invite staff to take responsibility for not only identifying, but also solving, problems that impede service to their customers. The key thing is to assert the goal of *solving* problems within their control, not just naming them. Too often, managers invite staff to develop a laundry list of complaints and the exercise stops there, with the manager feeling overwhelmed and overburdened and staff expecting actions on every problem they identified—actions on the part of others, not themselves.

Employee Input Meetings to Generate Improvements

Employee input meetings enable you to hear firsthand the suggestions and ideas your employees have about improvements that would remove or weaken barriers to impressive service. They also engage your team in making concrete improvements so that they can better serve customers.

Many people are reluctant to conduct this sort of meeting for fear it will degenerate into a complaint session. The following structure helps you to keep a clear focus on suggestions and improvements rather than complaints.

Method

1. Introduce the meeting by explaining, "The purpose of today's meeting is for us as a group to identify ways we can remove or weaken barriers that make it difficult to provide great service— service we provide to patients, their families, and any of our other customers."
2. Divide the group into small groups of three.
3. Assign two tasks:
   —Thinking about one customer group at a time, identify their frustrations with our service and list them on a big sheet of paper.
   —Now ask, "What would make our service better for our customers? In other words, What's one improvement that would really make a difference in our service quality—an improvement that is within our power?"
4. Tell your team that they will have just three minutes.
   Give them the following ground rules, which will allow this process to move along smoothly:
   —Be specific.
   —Don't blame; suggest instead.
   —Give each other a chance to talk.
   —Don't try to reach agreement.
5. After about three minutes, ask for the group's attention. Then ask them to contribute their suggestions as you record them on the flipchart. Push them to include suggestions on what they can do to tackle or alleviate the problem, not just what others or management can do.
6. After you have noted all of the suggestions together, sort them into categories such as "Quick-fix issues," "Needs work over time," and "Red tape–removal issues." Invite people to volunteer for a small committee that will review the lists and initiate efforts that involve staff in making the priority improvements. Make it clear that it will not be possible to solve all the problems or implement all of the improvements.
7. Thank the group for their input and thank them in advance for pursuing solutions to these problems.

Tips

- The way you listen and respond is critical. Accept everything employees say as legitimate in their eyes: don't judge, defend, argue, or resist anything an employee says.
- Use reflective listening. For example, "Sounds like you have good reasons to feel that way," or "I can see you feel very strongly about that," or "It's clear this has had a big effect on you!"
- Stay focused, listening in depth to what people are saying.
- Create a freewheeling atmosphere in which staff feel comfortable thinking of solutions. Don't let people critique every suggestion. Generate a bunch and then (and only then) ask people to focus on promising suggestions and to debug them so that they can work. If you critique people's ideas or let others do it, the flow of solutions will slow down tremendously.
- Engaging staff in solutions is easier said than done. Be sure to set a ground rule up front that staff will need to see some problems through to the end.
- To engage staff appropriately, help the group sort problems into those they can control and those they can't. Take responsibility for running interference on those they can't control, but you can.
- This kind of meeting should be a staple for your service. The ongoing understanding is "We identify problems and *share* responsibility for solving them—all for the sake of better service to our customers."

Develop Backup Plans Staff Can Use When Service Breaks Down

Sometimes things fall apart. Service breaks down. The system fails. It happens for reasons such as the following:

- Staff members don't show up and the shortage makes it impossible to serve customers.
- The one-and-only registration person becomes sick in the middle of a hectic day.
- Staff become consumed by difficult or complex customer situations.

- The computer crashes and patient appointments disappear from the system.
- The computer support person leaves early when a big project needs to get done. The computer crashes and no one knows what to do.
- The shuttle breaks down that takes patients back and forth to appointments between campuses.
- There's a flu epidemic and suddenly everyone wants a flu shot. The doctor's office has a ground swell of urgent calls.

The three F's take over: Staff become freaked, frustrated, and frantic. They switch into a crisis mode, during which it is difficult to develop rational alternatives to the emergency situation at hand. The best hope is to have *previously* developed backup systems or contingency plans, which some businesses call disaster plans. If you have disaster plans, when disaster strikes, people regroup and call forth their contingency plan for this kind of situation. They barely have to think.

For example, the doctor doesn't show up. A stream of customers has arrived and others are expected. A good disaster plan might include an on-call system for backup doctors in-house or at a neighboring service and transportation to get there. There should be a protocol for staff to use to apologize for the situation and offer options to the patient, including transportation to another doctor or a coupon for a free lunch and free transportation to their next appointment. The disaster plan would also include clarity about which other people in the service (or available by phone) can make rapid-fire phone calls to patients to cancel appointments later in the day.

While you probably can't prevent all unplanned crises from happening, you *can* work with staff to develop backup or disaster plans. The fact is, service doesn't have to break down if you have backup plans in place.

Undoubtedly, you and your team have some experience with *designed* ways to keep meeting customer needs despite service breakdowns. The challenge here is to develop backup plans for the remaining situations in which service breaks down to the detriment of the customer and the horror of staff.

Rx for Service Messes

This tool will help staff develop disaster plans for havoc-producing breakdowns in service that cannot be prevented.

Method

Hold a staff meeting in which you identify unpreventable service breakdowns and develop disaster plans.

1. Invite staff to share "Can you top this?" stories—real examples of times service fell apart to the extent that customer needs could not be served and staff became rattled by it.
2. After each story, ask staff to give a title to the story they just heard that describes the situation in a nutshell. For the earlier example, the story might have been "The Disappearing Doctor with Packed House," or "The Crammed Waiting Room, No Doctor" story. Write the titles on a board or flipchart page.
3. Refer staff to the famous quote from suffragist Susan B. Anthony, "Failure is impossible." Ask people to adopt this mind-set for the next 30 minutes: to pretend that service did not *have* to break down in the situations they described because they had backup plans to use when these situations arose.
4. Remind them that backup plans are not new to the team, and cite some you already have in place. For instance, do you already have a prearranged on-call system that designates backup caregivers when a caregiver doesn't show up? Do you have a backup system for staff coverage of phones when the receptionist becomes ill in the middle of the day or attends a training program or becomes otherwise unavailable? Do you have an established phone tree for use when someone needs to communicate an important message or instruction to all staff after hours? Give staff examples of backup plans they already use, as a reminder that they have some success with this kind of thinking.
5. Divide staff into small groups and assign each group a different service breakdown situation (from their list). Ask them to adopt the mind-set that failure is impossible and to develop a backup plan for the team to use when this situation occurs.
6. Give people this list of ideas as a resource. Challenge them to think outside the box and get creative with their solutions.

To Trigger Your Thinking about Backup Plans

- Would it help to designate a person who everyone knows will serve as the central command center when complex plans need to be enacted or coordinated?
- Would it help to line up *relief* people who can back up colleagues when they are, for any reason, unable to deliver service—in other words, a buddy system? A barter system of trading time with other services or departments? An on-call system? Regularly available temps that can be used for backup?
- Would it help to create incentives staff know they'll receive if they work harder and longer during crises: comp time, bonuses, free meals, the opportunity to dress casually, replacement time off, or the like?
- Would it help to figure out methods of support—ways colleagues can support people who are the only ones who can deliver services in a crisis situation? Can others figure out a way to help the people under fire feel taken care of during the crisis situation?
- Would it help to establish a signal for going into a confidential mode, a signal that means "Zip your lip about what's going on until the crisis is resolved"?
- Would it help to develop and have on hand scripts for staff to use when recurring service breakdowns occur, such as how to provide service despite a computer crash, or a protocol for how to communicate to a patient that they need to reschedule their appointment?

Get creative. Assume that Susan B. Anthony was right when she said, "Failure is impossible!"

7. After people have had a chance to work in teams on backup plans (in the meeting or between meetings), convene and share their proposals. Invite staff to cite the strengths of each proposal and suggest improvements. Send teams back to the drawing board to fine-tune their plans and write them down to be distributed to everyone and available when the crisis occurs next.
8. After the crisis occurs next, hold a debriefing to evaluate how the backup plan worked and make refinements again. Do what's needed to make a workable contingency plan for the specified situation.

Variations

- Ask people to identify impossible service situations instead of service messes. Then after brainstorming these impossible situations, challenge them to convert these from impossible to possible by thinking of creative contingency plans.
- Explain the goal and nature of contingency planning for service breakdowns. Ask people to brainstorm impossible situations. Then dare people who don't agree that these situations are impossible to volunteer to work on backup plans and present them for review at the next staff meeting. Or create a "failure is impossible" team or disaster planning squad and challenge them to create disaster plans to make it possible to deliver service in impossible situations.
- Challenge people to test the limits of their creativity. Ask them, "Imagine that every one of us could get a $100 personal bonus if we figured out a contingency plan that would enable us to meet customer needs when this disaster occurs."

Tips

- To make this work, *you* need to adopt the "failure is impossible attitude" first. Make sure you honestly want disaster plans that prevent in-crisis emotions from overtaking you and your staff. If you're thinking "Who wouldn't?" think again. Many managers thrive on swooping in like a superhero to solve crisis situations after the fact. For them, this can be very exciting and give them a sense of indispensability. When you have a disaster plan, it's different. You can actually maintain a sense of calm and business as usual when disaster strikes, because people know what to do and they do it. The opportunities for manager as superhero diminish.
- When staff develop disaster plans that seem workable, devote time to having coworkers debug these plans and work out the details, so that there is great clarity about how to enact the plan when the time comes.

Change gears now. If you used the above tools, you probably have some victories to show for your team. The next section looks at ways to appreciate these before chasing after the next problem.

Stop to Smell the Roses

When you use these tools with staff to identify and tackle barriers to service delivery, you are definitely going to make improvements happen. And *that* is a cause for celebration, or at least to stop to savor your successes. Use these tools to help staff recognize their accomplishments in removing barriers before they rush on to remove others. If you don't stop to appreciate the improvements you've made, people feel that the problems are endless and unrelenting.

Three Things

This tool helps staff focus on those things that are working or improving—a refreshing break from focusing on problem after problem.

Method

1. Post these questions around the room on flipchart pages:

Three Things

- What are three things that are getting easier for me to do?
- What are three things I'm enjoying doing?
- What are three ways I think we're making a difference to our customers?
- What are three ways we're working well as a team?

---

2. Have staff write one or two responses for each topic on Post-Its and then go around and stick them onto the right flipcharts.
3. Have people mill around to read everyone's contributions.
4. Afterward, ask people to identify common themes and service barriers they would like to tackle so that they can see progress on those listed on these charts the next time they do this activity.

Variation

- To identify patterns and themes and summarize the findings, consider forming four small groups. Have each group cluster around one flipchart to analyze what's there and prepare to report back to the larger group the most common answers, the most surprising answers, and the answers you hope to see next time.

Tips

- Be sure to give everyone a chance to talk. Don't let a select few dominate the process.
- The wrap-up for this activity is important. You want people to think about the service features, problems, or behaviors that they want to crack in the next month, so it will appear as progress on these charts the next time around.

Against the Odds

This tool helps you to appreciate the motivation and talent of people dedicated to tackling *difficult* barriers and improvements.

Method

1. Pass out this worksheet and give people a chance to fill out answers to as many questions as they can.

Against the Odds

In the last month:

A barrier I helped to remove for the sake of our customers was

_____.

Something good I made happen for customers because I got creative was _____.

Something good I made happen for customers because I took a risk was _____.

Something good I made happen for customers because I pushed the limits was _____.

A way others supported me was _____.

2. After people have filled in what they can, form a circle and, one topic at a time, ask people to go around and give their answers, passing if they have no answer. Encourage listening and mutual appreciation.

3. At the end, congratulate people on the improvements they helped to make, and also on the personal courage, creativity, and focus it took to make these improvements.

Tips

• Participate yourself, so you can also share your contributions to removing barriers. This is a great way to show that you've been working on removing those barriers that you uniquely need to address in your management role as well as those you helped to address along with team members.

• Make a short pitch up front that encourages people to tell all— and not to be bashful. Say, "We are so busy, and move from problem to problem so fast, that we sometimes miss seeing what people did that created the improvements we're making. This is the time to slow down and notice all of the important effort, creativity, and courage people applied to improving service for our customers."

Conclusion

Although there's a lot involved in removing the barriers that prevent staff from meeting customer needs, every bit of improvement produces payoffs for staff and customers. One of the criticisms of the quality management process is that lots of energy is going into the big systems that impact many customers and many departments, but people don't seem to focus on the smaller things that trip people up everyday—the everyday nuisances and frustrations. Here's your chance. And you don't need to use fancy tools, processes, or facilitators. Just start somewhere! Work on one area at a time and reap the benefits. You'll find that, as soon as people experience positive results, they'll have renewed energy and enthusiasm for continuing the process.

Chapter 5

• • •

Reduce Anxiety to Increase Satisfaction

Do You Need to Read This Chapter?

Riddle: What do all of these situations have in common?

- Waiting for your appointment
- Finding a parking space
- Worrying about being on time
- Answering questions about insurance
- Waiting in the waiting room
- Disrobing in the changing room
- Hearing the noise of the MRI machine
- Making the trip to the doctor's office
- Anticipating news while the doctor examines you
- Waiting for the baby-sitter
- Being asked the same questions by the receptionist, then the nurse
- Watching the doctor prepare to take your blood pressure
- Sitting in the waiting room next to someone coughing

The answer: They all cause patients to feel *anxiety* about their medical appointments and procedures. Among patients, anxiety runs amok. If you've witnessed anxiety among the patients you serve, this chapter is for you. Anxiety reduction is a powerful approach to increasing patient satisfaction. It matters a great deal to patients. And it is an angle on service improvement that staff can easily understand and embrace.

Written especially for doctors' offices and ambulatory care (but also applicable to inpatient or residential settings), this chapter introduces the concept of anxiety reduction and offers a four-step process with which you and your staff can reduce anxiety among patients.

A Case for the Anxiety Reduction Approach

As you know, growth in primary care and ambulatory care and the decline of inpatient volume have been dramatic. These trends have come so quickly that they have propelled hospitals to make wrenching decisions about services, staffing, programs, and systems. Personnel have been transferred, hurriedly cross-trained, or laid off to meet the demands of the mushrooming outpatient and shrinking inpatient markets.

If you're a service or product line manager or a physician leader, you won't find much guidance to navigate the new ambulatory care environment. You won't find much about how to enhance patient or member satisfaction from senior managers, books, or consultants. The inpatient market has consumed most health care resources.

Until now, most research on patient satisfaction has been sponsored by hospitals and has thus focused on the inpatient's experience, with disproportionately little attention to outpatient satisfaction and the factors that influence it. The scarcity of research on patient satisfaction with ambulatory care is aggravated by the fact that such research is hard to do because of the variety of ambulatory care services. Ambulatory care is actually a portfolio of many different businesses, which raises questions about the extent to which you can generalize research findings from one service to others.

The lion's share of health care services are delivered in doctors' offices and other ambulatory care settings. With ambulatory care skyrocketing, so have efforts to gain a competitive edge by gaining a service advantage. Managed care companies now shop for providers who not only keep their costs low, but also promise positive clinical outcomes and high levels of patient satisfaction.

Groundbreaking Research Provides the Key

Elizabeth Dunn, Carmhiel Brown, and Barry Love of the marketing department of Thomas Jefferson University Hospital in Philadelphia saw the burgeoning growth of outpatient care and were undaunted by the difficulties inherent in studying patient satisfaction in *diverse* ambulatory care settings. In 1994 they conducted a qualitative study to identify the factors that affect patient satisfaction in *ambulatory care* settings.[1] Their ultimate purpose was to understand the ambulatory care experience from the patient's perspective and to identify commonalities in experience that cut across a wide variety of outpatient procedures and services. Ultimately, their findings have far-reaching implications for heightening patient satisfaction in many, if not all, health care settings.

With the help of the Omega Group, Inc., in Haverford, Pennsylvania, Jefferson Hospital marketers conducted in-depth personal interviews with 12 consumers who had recent outpatient experiences in various Philadelphia-area hospitals. These patients had experienced many services, including outpatient surgery, advanced diagnostic cardiac testing, and imaging services. The study's objectives were to understand the outpatient experience from the patient's perspective and to identify commonalities across a wide variety of services—commonalities that would suggest service improvement opportunities. Questions probed patients' experiences and their evaluations of those experiences. Also, a guided visualization technique was used to help consumers picture and describe in graphic detail experiences with outpatient care that particularly satisfied or upset them.

This study yielded one clear and powerful conclusion: No matter what the content and purpose of care, the dominant experience for the patient was *anxiety.* Throughout the interviews, respondents used words like *tense, nervous, anxious, apprehensive, scared, hesitant, alone,* and *abandoned* to describe their emotional states—all words associated with anxiety.

Patient anxiety matters to health care professionals because it has many negative consequences for patients:

- Anxiety impairs their attention.
- Anxiety drives people to seek comfort and security, which explains why patients so greatly appreciate small comfort-giving gestures on the part of caregivers.
- Anxiety lowers frustration tolerance, which is why caregivers perceive patients as irritable.
- Anxiety interferes with memory and retention of information, and therefore compliance. This leads patients to call caregivers and ask, "Now what did you say I was supposed to do?"
- Anxiety reduces people's ability to handle ambiguity, choices, and problem solving. It interferes with rational thinking.
- Anxiety increases people's perception of pain.

Patients described anxiety at many specific points before, during, and after receiving the service. It started with someone telling them that they needed a visit, test, or procedure and ended with the patient waiting at home for results. Furthermore, Dunn et al. found that the anxiety was cumulative. For some, anxiety began at the care-giver's office when the procedure was ordered, and it accumulated as the patient proceeded through each step of the experience. By the time the patient arrived for the procedure itself, he or she had been collect-ing anxiety for days or even weeks. A person who became anxious when looking for a parking space at the doctor's office became even more anxious when she had to wait, and even more anxious when the doctor was taking her blood pressure. According to patients, the anx-ieties piled up, one upon the other, instead of peaking and dissipating. By the time a patient was ready to leave the office, he or she was often exhausted from the increasing level of anxiety and stress of proceed-ing through the health care experience.

The Effects of Anxiety on Customer Service

Anxiety can create a downward spiral for patients with effects on caregivers, too. By the time patients arrive for a doctor's appointment, they have been anxious about the visit and the results for days or weeks. Their stress has increased during the appointment scheduling and travel to the appointment. They're not only worried about their physical health, but also about the pain or embarrassment associated with the physical exam. All this is happening when they arrive.

It's no wonder that the patient seems *unreasonably* annoyed when the receptionist doesn't make eye contact. The receptionist asks the patient to complete the form, and the patient, because of reduced abil-ity to concentrate, fills out the form incorrectly or interrupts the recep-tionist to ask questions. Because the receptionist is very busy, he or she shows annoyance with the patient in subtle ways. Because of the patient's heightened sensitivity, the patient senses these cues and becomes even more irritable or upset—all this before the patient even sits down to endure what they expect will be an indefinite wait.

What's the punch line (as if it isn't obvious)? As caregivers, we can increase the satisfaction of people seeking health care by focus-ing on preventing or reducing their anxiety. If patients see that we are going above and beyond to prevent or reduce their anxiety, they are more than satisfied. They are impressed and grateful—two feel-ings that, in combination, are keys to patient loyalty.

If you run an ambulatory care service or medical practice, anxiety reduction offers you a simple, doable, and understandable driver of service improvement. All staff and patients understand anxiety and stress. When you ask people, "What increases your anxiety?" they can tell you. When you ask staff to identify patient anxiety, they can because of their own ample experience. When you ask people to develop ways to reduce anxiety in others, they can usually think of ways to do this.

But, say some, patients are irrational about their health care. There's only so much you can do to make them rational. We're not trying to make them rational. That's not the point. The point is that health care (including yours no doubt) is very, very personal and leaves people feeling very, very vulnerable. As humanistic people, why not respect that fact and do what we can to cushion the inevitable stresses related to patient health care? Providers shouldn't add insult to injury but should instead create a nurturing environment for people in highly stressful situations.

Make anxiety reduction for patients and families a single overarching focus for service improvement in your medical practice or other ambulatory care setting. If you're from an inpatient setting, consider it, too. While the Jefferson research focused on outpatients, the same approach makes sense for any service, outpatient or inpatient, nursing homes, home care, acute care, or any health care. Staff understand it and can describe it to others. Patients and their families perceive it and appreciate it. It's a win-win strategy.

A Simple Approach

If you think the research finding of anxiety reduction as the key to service improvement is a no-brainer, you'll be happy to know that the strategy for decreasing patient anxiety is not hard at all. The process we describe here involves staff in ways that they are likely to enjoy, and that means you won't have to do this strategy all by yourself or against their will.

Use this four-step process:

Step 1: Map patient pathways through your service.
Step 2: Pinpoint anxiety points.
Step 3: Remedy with prevention and anxiety reduction strategies.
Step 4: Check satisfaction and make further improvements.

Map Patient Pathways through Your Service

Engage staff in breaking down your service into the steps a *patient* takes through it—from their perspective. Here's an example from the Jefferson study of the typical steps through an outpatient procedure:

Patients' Pathway through an Outpatient Procedure

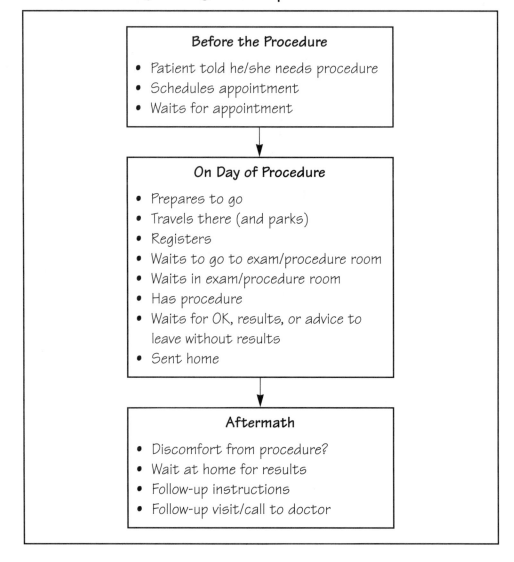

Before the Procedure

- Patient told he/she needs procedure
- Schedules appointment
- Waits for appointment

On Day of Procedure

- Prepares to go
- Travels there (and parks)
- Registers
- Waits to go to exam/procedure room
- Waits in exam/procedure room
- Has procedure
- Waits for OK, results, or advice to leave without results
- Sent home

Aftermath

- Discomfort from procedure?
- Wait at home for results
- Follow-up instructions
- Follow-up visit/call to doctor

Patient Shadowing to Produce Patient Pathways

This tool aids in mapping the steps through your service from the patient's perspective, so you can identify anxiety points in a systematic fashion.

Method

1. Categorize your patients into service categories according to their purpose for using your office or service. Determine which patients follow roughly the same pathway through your services. Be sure to create a category for the highest volume uses of your service—for example, patients who come for a checkup or patients who come for a particular procedure.

2. For each service category, arrange for two staff members to shadow two different patients through the service (asking the patients' permission up front of course). The staff shadow's job is to see the service from the patient's perspective and jot down the sequence of events from the patient's point of view. Where do they go first, then where, then where, and descriptively—not evaluatively—what happens at each point?

3. Have the two staff shadows get together and agree on a patient pathway. Ask them to draw the patient's pathway through the service, pinpointing each step along the way—then put this in a form that a patient can look at and understand.

4. Have the two staff shadows present their findings at a staff meeting, giving others a chance to react and fine-tune.

 Tips

• Yes, it's really a flowchart, but very often staff think of flowcharts as the map of our work processes and systems from the *provider's* perspective, not the *patient's* perspective. So, call it something else, like *patient pathway*.

• Have the shadows do their work during one week, so it doesn't take up too much time.

• Urge them to be descriptive (as if they are making a movie of the service), not evaluative, interpretive, or judgmental.

Pinpoint Anxiety Points

With the patient pathways in hand, consult patients and their families to identify where along the pathways they feel anxiety or stress and why (and while you're at it, ask what would help).

Personal Interviews with Former Patients and Their Families

Personal interviews will show you when, where, and why patients feel anxiety on the pathway through your service, so you'll know which anxiety points to fix or relieve.

Method

1. Identify skilled interviewers available to you (such as patient relations or marketing professionals, if your organization has access to such people, or outside consultants) or use staff members who can listen nondefensively.
2. Convene the interviewers and orient them to the purpose of the interviews and how to conduct them. Here's a sample script and question guide for them to use. Provide practice and preparation time, and answer their questions.

Sample Script for Use in Interviews

We are involved in an effort to improve our services for the sake of our patients. To do this, we want to learn more about when our patients and their families feel stressed or anxious during their experiences with us, so that we can make changes that reduce their anxiety and stress. I'm asking your help. Will you talk about your experience with us and let me ask you a few questions about it? I promise to keep what you say confidential. After I interview several people, I'll summarize the results without mentioning any names. No one will know what any specific person said. Also, I'd like to take notes so I don't forget anything you say. Is this all right with you? Great. This will be a big help to us as we work on improving our services.

Question guide:

1. What has been your most satisfying health care experience outside of hospitals—for instance, in a doctor's office or other ambulatory care setting? What made it so?
2. What do you recall as your most disturbing or upsetting health care experience outside of a hospital? What made it so?
3. What is important to you in a health care experience? What should happen? What shouldn't happen?
4. I'd like to learn more from you about one of your experiences with us, when you came to us for _____. Do you recall that time? Tell me about it.

Now, as I see it, there were many steps you went through in that experience. Some parts of your experience happened before you came to our building; others happened once you got here, and continued after you went home. I'd appreciate if you would tell me what your experience was like before, during, and after your visit. [For each time period, first ask open questions that invite people to talk about whatever pops into their minds. Then and only then, ask about stress or anxiety they felt at specific steps along the pathway.]

Let's start with before your visit:

5. What was your experience like with us once you decided to have an appointment, but before you came here?
6. Did you feel any anxiety or stress before your appointment?
7. What did you think and what did you feel?
8. Why?
9. Is there anything we could have done to relieve or prevent that?

[Then, focus on each step in the patient's pathway and ask the following:]

10. Specifically, were there any problems or did you feel any stress or anxiety when _____ [for example, you talked with our scheduler and made your appointment].
11. What was the problem or stress you felt?
12. Why?
13. Is there anything we could have done to relieve or prevent that stress or anxiety?

[Do this same series of questions for previsit, during visit, and postvisit steps in pathway.]

3. After the interviews, have interviewers get together to process their results. For every step in each pathway, they need to pinpoint the most frequently mentioned anxiety or stress points. Also, for use in the next step of this process, they need to collate the ideas patients offered for remedying or easing these stress/anxiety points. It's helpful to summarize results in the form of an addendum to the patient pathway chart developed above. Here's an example of such a summary chart from the Jefferson study:[2]

Anxiety Related to the Outpatient Procedure

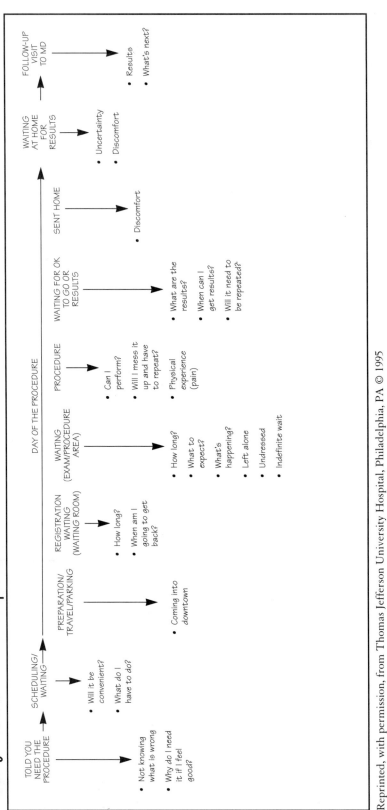

Reprinted, with permission, from Thomas Jefferson University Hospital, Philadelphia, PA © 1995

—Stress point 1: In the physician's office, when the patient is first told that he or she needs an outpatient procedure, the patient's anxiety stems from concern about what is wrong. They often feel the disorienting sensation of "Why do I need a test if I feel good?" and "Can I trust my body to tell me if I'm healthy?"

—Stress point 2: Scheduling and waiting for the procedure
  –"Will I have to wait and keep feeling worried? Will I be able to get off from work? Will I be able to arrange child care? What about transportation?"

—Stress point 3: Preparing for the scheduled appointment
  –"Do I have to fast and have hunger increase my discomfort? Will I have to undergo some strange or uncomfortable procedure, such as an enema or drinking a terrible-tasting substance? Will I be clean enough? Will doctors and nurses think I have an unusual-looking body?"

—Stress point 4: Travel and parking
  –"Will I find a parking space? Will I find my way to the exact service location? What if I get lost? Will someone be there to help me? Will they still take me if I'm late?"

—Stress point 5: Registration and waiting in the outer office
  –"Will I remember and be able to write down the information they need from me? Will I have to wait endlessly? Will I get back to work on time? Will I get a parking ticket?"

—Stress point 6: The procedure waiting room
  –"Will it hurt? Will I be able to perform adequately? Can I be still? Will I cry out?"

—Stress point 7: The procedure
  –"What does that scary equipment do to me? Will it work? Will they have to do it again?"

—Stress point 8: Waiting
  –"Do I have to wait for the results? Is it OK for me to go home?"

—Stress point 9: After the patient leaves
  –"What are the results? What does this mean to me? Will I have to go back? Will I remember to take my medicine? What next?"

Tips

- Although this process is tedious, it produces the rich, specific results you need in order to identify priority areas for service improvement by way of anxiety reduction.

- Discuss with your staff the word *anxiety*. Several issues might arise over use of this word. Ask staff what their issues are with the word and talk these through. For instance, some people see anxiety as pathological. Help staff to see it instead as an inevitable, normal feeling. If it works better for them, encourage them to use the word *stress* instead. Help them adopt the attitude that it's OK for people to feel anxious or stressed; it's not a negative thing. Also, some staff might rightly be concerned that some customers might feel embarrassed if caught showing anxiety and might balk a little if staff show empathy for this. Suggest to staff that they be sensitive to labeling customers as anxious if the customer shows any annoyance or resistance when staff say such things as "I can understand that this makes you anxious." Discuss these and other possible issues staff have with the word *anxiety*.

- Why use personal interviews with patients? They afford greater depth of questioning and disclosure. You'll learn more. Can they be done by phone? Yes, but in person works better.

- Don't divide up interview assignments by service category. Have each interviewer interview people in each service category, so that when the interviewers get together to process their results, they will benefit from multiple perspectives on each patient pathway.

- Doctors' offices and small services might want to conduct focus groups periodically instead of doing personal interviews, which consume more time. Although a focus group doesn't work quite as well—because you need to probe for the details to really learn a lot about patients' anxiety at specific steps in your processes—use focus groups if you don't have the staff to do personal interviews. The results are valuable and will give you substantial material for follow up. They just aren't as rich or detailed because there is less time per person to probe for remedies.

Remedy with Prevention and Anxiety Reduction Strategies

With anxiety points associated with your service pathways in hand, work on remedies of two sorts: Remedies that prevent predictable anxiety, and remedies that ease unpreventable anxieties. For instance, an example of a preventable stress point is this: If your patients get anxious trying to find your location, send them a map with landmarks ahead of time—before they have to ask. An example of an unpreventable stress point is this: If patients perceive even a brief waiting time as interminable, institute a standard whereby a designated staff member touches base with the patient at least every ten minutes with an accurate, honest update on the expected wait that remains. And supply the patient with magazines and a fish tank to look at to make the time *feel* like it's going faster. Once you identify the stress points, staff will find it easy to figure out ways to reduce stress at each point.

Use the following tool to create formats for staff or subcommittee meetings.

Meeting to Generate Remedies

This tool has two purposes:

1. To identify ways to prevent patient anxiety at specific points along the pathway through your practice or service
2. To identify ways to ease anxiety that cannot be prevented

Method

1. Organize your team into subteams (or if small, use the whole team).
2. At team meetings, use this simple format for generating remedies for patient and family anxieties associated with your services.
3. For one patient pathway at a time do the following:
   —Show summary chart of the main anxiety/stress points.
   —Focusing on one at a time, invite staff to brainstorm in response to two questions:

–What, if anything, can we possibly do to prevent this anxiety in the first place?

–If we didn't or can't prevent it, how could we ease it once it has occurred?

4. Use a chart or flipchart page formatted like this to guide the discussion:

Anxiety Points

Preventable Types of Anxiety	
Anxiety Point	Prevention Ideas
Finding way there	• Send map • Call and offer help • Send someone to pick up patient
Unpreventable Types of Anxiety	
Anxiety point	Ideas for easing anxiety
Worrying about procedure	• Give explanation of when you'll feel what—ahead of time • Offer name of someone to talk to who has had procedure • Offer option of relaxer medicine

5. For each brainstormed list, ask people individually to look over the list and pick three ideas that they think have the greatest potential to prevent (or ease) the anxiety. Vote and see if there's convergence on a few ideas.

6. Decide together how to follow up on these ideas. Do they need more discussion? Can some one person investigate further or run with the ball? Does a team need to work out the details? Clearly decide on the next steps for each high-potential idea.

7. Agree on a time when people will report back the status of their follow-up.

Variations

- In a large practice or service where there are groups of people in the same roles, subdivide anxiety points into categories based on the staff group in whose domain the anxieties occur. For instance, imagine a radiology or imaging service. Patient categories might be inpatients, outpatients, or patients by machine type, but all these patients might interact with the same staff. For instance, patients in all categories might see receptionists, some might all see nuclear medicine technologists, and so on. In this case, cluster all the anxiety points that fall within the domain of receptionists and have receptionists work on remedies for those, and do the same for technologists. Have them work on all of the anxiety points (for all patient types) that fall within their domain of activity.
- Focus on one anxiety point at each staff meeting. Invite staff to brainstorm ways to relieve or prevent patient anxiety at that point.
- Create a patient anxiety reduction fund. Develop a subcommittee to establish criteria for receiving money from the fund and put that group in charge of dispensing the fund in response to proposals. Some anxiety reduction interventions cost a few dollars.
- Create and support user groups of patients to help you identify and remedy anxieties. You can also create an anti-hassle brigade or patient comfort team or other cleverly named teams to stamp out preventable causes of patient anxiety.

Tips

- Although meetings encourage cross-fertilization of ideas, supplement them with suggestion boxes, bulletin boards, and contests in which you focus on one anxiety at a time and invite people to submit their great ideas for relieving or preventing the anxiety.
- If your service is big enough, involve staff in helping to produce remedies not only for their own service/practice, but also for other people's. They often bring fresher perspectives and ideas to other people's services.

Check Satisfaction and Make Further Improvements

Once you institute improvements, monitor the results and also keep the door open to identify additional anxiety points and remedies.

Feedback Device Aligned with Pathway

This tool will help you to collect feedback about each step along patients' pathways so you can determine how you're doing at preventing or relieving the anxiety you intended to alleviate and can identify further opportunities for improvement.

Method
Realign your satisfaction survey methods with your work on anxiety reduction.

1. Add this wonderful overall question: "To what extent did staff take steps to relieve your anxiety and stress?" Research at Jefferson showed that this question is highly correlated with patients' overall satisfaction.
2. Also, develop a more specific survey that provides you with feedback about your efforts to reduce anxiety at each point along the patient's pathway through your practice/service. Focus questions on the extent to which the patient thought your staff succeeded or didn't succeed in preventing or easing anxiety at each point. Do it in a straightforward fashion. Also ask for patient assessments of specific remedies. For instance, consider this satisfaction tool developed for physician customers of the Albert Einstein Medical Center's admitting service. It was built along the same principles: Identify the steps in their pathway through the service; identify their anxiety points; and take steps to relieve these anxieties through terrific service. This survey—aligned with physicians' anxiety points in each phase of the admitting department's service pathway—monitors ongoing effectiveness of the department's service improvement efforts and pinpoints anxiety points that warrant further attention.

Admissions Survey

Based on discussions with our physician customers, we outlined the sequence of admitting services that impact most on physicians (organized around anxiety points).

For each activity, we identified physicians' key requirements or expectations. Please evaluate how you perceive the admitting process in relation to each of these items:

		Poor				Excellent
Reservations	• Access to reservations/scheduling	1	2	3	4	5
	• Ease of providing information requested	1	2	3	4	5
	• Courtesy of the reservation staff	1	2	3	4	5
Preadmission Testing	• Ease of scheduling	1	2	3	4	5
	• Courtesy of scheduling staff	1	2	3	4	5
	• Chart completion and result coordination	1	2	3	4	5
	• Nurse communication to physicians about abnormal results	1	2	3	4	5
	• Courtesy of nurse	1	2	3	4	5
Financial Clearance	• Timeliness of insurance verification	1	2	3	4	5
	• Communication to physician of insurance problems	1	2	3	4	5
	• Courtesy of financial counseling staff	1	2	3	4	5
Precertification	• Helpfulness of having the hospital perform this service	1	2	3	4	5
	• Communications between precert nurse and physician/physician office	1	2	3	4	5
	• Courtesy of nurses	1	2	3	4	5
Bed Assignment	• Timeliness of bed availability	1	2	3	4	5
	• Appropriateness of bed assignments	1	2	3	4	5
	• Courtesy of "bed board" staff	1	2	3	4	5
	• Courtesy of nurse facilitators	1	2	3	4	5

Variation

- Also consider doing a quarterly interview study in which you obtain once again in-depth information from patients about anxiety points during your services.

 Tips

- Once you align your feedback methods with your anxiety reduction work, be sure to plan for a feedback loop to staff, so they see the results, which in turn spark further thinking about service improvements.
- Also build attention to anxiety reduction into everyday life. Coach staff to ask patients face-to-face *during* the service, "Is there anything I can do for you to reduce your concern or anxiety about this?"

Variations in Your Approach to Anxiety Reduction

- Consider helping staff tune into and notice patient anxiety. Help staff identify the signs of anxiety, so that they take a deep breath and think of things they can do right there to intervene with the patient—behaviors that help the patient ask questions, help the patient to explain, offer comfort and options, and the like. Accomplish this awareness raising about the signs of anxiety by reviewing case situations in staff meetings or by securing training for staff on verbal and nonverbal listening.
- Consider also focusing on known anxiety points and how to relieve them. For instance, it is well known that patients become anxious when they enter a health care facility, when they complain to a health care provider, and when they are hearing a health care worker explain something important to them that they need to retain. The book *Service Savvy Health Care: One Goal at a Time* (W. Leebov, S. Afriat, and J. Presha; AHA Press, 1998) provides strategies for tackling these well-known anxiety points one at a time. The book includes a do-it-yourself kit for improving staff greetings of customers throughout your service, to reduce their anxiety and make them feel welcome and noticed. Another do-it-yourself kit shows how to improve service recovery or complaint handling by staff. A third do-it-

yourself kit describes how staff can provide effective explanations and inform patients so well that they give them confidence and stem the tide of their anxiety. Tackle one well-known source of anxiety (for example, greetings, explanations, confidentiality, privacy, long waits, and the like) one goal at a time.

- The same processes described here work for any customer group, not just patients and families. If the customers you want to satisfy are internal customers or managed care company staff or physicians, use the same process. Identify their pathways through your services and their main anxiety points along the pathways. Develop remedies and monitor how well these remedies are working.

    —For example, let's say you run a housekeeping department in a hospital. Find out the anxiety points patients have about your cleaning services. Do they get anxious not knowing when a housekeeper is coming? Do they get anxious wondering if the housekeeper will wake them up after a bad night of sleep? Do they get anxious wondering if the cleaning fluids' odor will cause them nausea? Do they get anxious because of embarrassment over messing up the sheets? After staff conduct interviews to find out people's anxiety points, they can brainstorm ways to avoid preventable sources of anxiety and ease unpreventable ones. If patients get anxious because of embarrassment over messing up sheets, the housekeepers can be prepared with words that ease that anxiety, such as, "Oh, this happens when you're a patient. I know you can't help it. And I deal with it all the time, and it doesn't bother me a bit." If patients worry that staff will wake them up, on the first day of care, the housekeeper should drop in when the patient is awake and tell the patient that they will be careful not to do this.

    —Another example is the managed care company as customer: Have staff interview the people from the company with whom they interact and find out what creates stress for them when dealing with this service. Do they feel stressed trying to get answers by a certain time of day? Do they get stressed because they can't count on receiving follow-up calls by a certain time? Again, once the stress points are identified, staff can think of methods for easing them. The same approach works and is an easy, straightforward approach to service improvement and customer satisfaction.

Objections to the Anxiety Reduction Process

Here are some of the questions and reservations people have expressed to us when introduced to the anxiety reduction process, and our responses:

Isn't Anxiety Inevitable When You're Talking about People's Health and Health Care?

Absolutely. But all the more reason to take steps to decrease it. People expect to feel anxious, and they are grateful when you show you care enough to minimize their anxiety through your own proactive efforts.

What about Staff Anxiety? Doesn't That Count, Too?

Staff anxiety certainly gets in the way of serving patients, and serving patients is the job. So, staff anxiety is also a concern. Why not try the same approach (identify anxiety points and brainstorm and install remedies) in response to staff anxieties? This would be a great complement to the similar work done to relieve patient anxieties. Two other chapters in this book can help you here: chapter 4, "Remove Barriers so Staff Can Serve Customers," and chapter 6, "Help Staff Cope Better in a Stressful Atmosphere."

This Approach Is Qualitative and Doesn't Seem Very Scientific.

It is qualitative, but ask yourself, "Is it face valid? Does it make sense?" You will probably agree that it does. Patients are plagued by anxiety just as staff are plagued by stress. If you take steps to relieve it, patients will be grateful, more satisfied, and even impressed. It's that simple.

Isn't This Approach Obvious?

Yes, it's obvious that people will feel better about your service if you don't make them any more anxious than they already are when they are already feeling sensitive and vulnerable. But ask yourself, "Why have we made service improvement so difficult and complex? Why haven't we just adopted the approach of asking, 'How can we reduce people's anxiety so they aren't so nervous, worried, panicked, and irritable when receiving our services?' Why haven't we adopted this straightforward approach already if it's so obvious?" We'll agree that it's obvious once everyone is instinctively doing it.

Conclusion

Using anxiety reduction as the driver for service improvement is simple and accessible. Show us a health care worker who wants to *increase* the stress patients feel. That's not why people become health care professionals. They want to have positive effects on people's well-being. Efforts to decrease anxiety make sense and do not tend to breed staff resistance. Staff share the goal of satisfying patients, and they also know that the anxiety-free patient makes their life at work much easier.

Improvements can be made one service at a time, one patient pathway at a time—in fact, one anxiety point at a time. And because anxiety has a cumulative effect, one anxiety piles onto the next, creating an increasing negative impact. Why not chip away at anxiety points one at a time for a cumulative positive impact?

References and Related Resources

1. Elizabeth Dunn, Carmhiel Brown, and Barry Love, "Decreasing Anxiety," *Journal of Healthcare Marketing* 15, no. 1 (spring 1995).

2. Dunn, Carmhiel, and Love, "Decreasing Anxiety."

Carmhiel Brown, Marketing Department, Jefferson Health System, 11th and Walnut Streets, Philadelphia, PA 19107.

Elizabeth Dunn Associates, 321 Queen Street, Philadelphia, PA 19147.

Wendy Leebov, Susan Afriat, and Jeanne Presha, *Service Savvy Health Care: One Goal at a Time* (Chicago: AHA Press, 1998).

Barry Love, Omega Group, Inc., 600 Haverford Road, Suite 100, Haverford, PA 19041.

Chapter 6

• • •

Help Staff Cope Better in a Stressful Atmosphere

Do You Need to Read This Chapter?

Answer the following questions related to how your staff handle stress:

- Do some people on the team blame others for mistakes and problems with customers?
- Do staff members engage in backbiting and finger-pointing?
- Do people seem tired and find demanding customers exhausting?
- Do people complain about not being appreciated?
- Do people seem unable to see even obvious solutions when presented with tasks or problems?
- Does there seem to be a contagious negativism within the team?
- Are staff less flexible than they used to be when changes occur?
- Do staff come in late and call in sick more than they used to?
- Do staff talk every day about being under tremendous pressure and stress?
- Do staff members sometimes lose it in front of customers?

If the majority of your answers are yes, then your team members are showing signs of stress that are interfering with their ability to deliver great service to their customers. This chapter is designed to help you create a more nurturing environment for your team, an environment that fosters vitality, resilience, and mutual support among stressed service workers. It will show you how to help your staff develop coping skills to maintain the personal reserves needed to give customers their energy, attention, and positive regard.

Stress Strangles Service

You know this. People pass on their feelings to others. When people on your team feel good, they pass on these feelings to customers. When people on your team feel bad, they pass on these feelings, too. When staff feel stressed, out of control, upset, exhausted, or frazzled, this depletes them and hurts their productivity and the quality of service they're able to extend to customers and to each other. They don't give as much to customers; they aren't as supportive of coworkers; they can't solve problems creatively; and they tend not to take good care of themselves, causing them to be more prone to illness.

The solutions are not easy because most of us in health care don't have the resources to remove the sources of stress. We can't add staff we can't afford. And we can't simply remove the pressures staff feel as operators in the current health care system. We can't say, "Too many paperwork demands? No problem! Stop doing it." We can't say, "At the end of your rope because you're hanging on the phone endlessly waiting for approvals from a managed care company? No problem. Hang up!" We can't say, "Hassled by customers who are upset because they have to wait so long for an appointment? No problem. Give them one for today." We can't say, "Irritable because coworkers are taking out their stress on you? No problem. Avoid them. Don't work with them anymore!" We can't say, "Rattled and insecure because of so much change? No problem. We'll slow things down and let others change, not us!"

We can't say any of these things because they are, in many of our settings, artifacts of our current health care system. Although heads of services might be talking to staff about the wonderful opportunities presented by the changes occurring in health care and in their organization, most people working on the front line aren't having much fun. They are experiencing work that is difficult and demanding, physically and emotionally.

What Can You Do?

Plenty! Although you can't remove many of the sources of stress, you have the power to alter for the better your work team's dynamics. These dynamics can aggravate the stress and pain, or they can help employees feel support, encouragement, and care in spite of the demands, expectations, and changes that press on them. You can help to make your work environment a place where problems are nipped in the bud, where staff feel "We're in this together." You can help staff learn to support, not aggravate, each other through particularly harrowing moments. You can help staff learn new ways to respond to difficult situations, so they don't get caught up in a spiral of negativity. You can help staff feel valued and appreciated for the hard work they're doing and the quality of service they're extending to others despite the pressures on them.

Realistically, how can you do this in today's crazy health care world? First of all, you can't do it *for* employees. You have to do it *with* them—or, better yet, help them do it for themselves. Employees need to take full responsibility for creating and maintaining an environment that nurtures them in their difficult, stressed roles. Second, you can't help by protecting or mothering employees, either. You can't lessen the load, take jobs away, stop changes from impinging on employees, or turn back the clock so things are as they used to be.

But you can do a great deal to create a place where employees can be more successful and more gratified in their work, where they can learn and grow, and where they recognize and deal better with the stresses their coworkers and customers are under.

A Three-Pronged Prescription

Pick the approaches that you think will work best for your team:

1. Help staff make work-space improvements that reduce stress and nurture them better. Involve staff in taking responsibility for creating a work space that fosters calmness, efficiency, and comfort.
2. Help staff develop personal coping skills sorely needed when working in a high-stress environment; in other words, help staff take better care of themselves during times of stress.

3. Build a supportive team so that people work more effectively with strained coworkers and avoid getting drawn into the downward spiral of negativity themselves. Help staff develop a shared vision of a supportive work team and then institute ways they can translate that vision into reality.

Approach 1: Help Staff Make Work-Space Improvements for Greater Calm, Efficiency, and Comfort

Shut your eyes and see if you can envision your own work space. Are the sounds you hear harsh or soothing? Are the colors warm or cold, easy on the eyes or glaring? Do you feel cramped because of furniture and files that are too close to you or hanging overhead? Is there disarray that gives you a feeling of being scattered and out of control? If you were to walk into that space and just sit down, what feelings would the space engender?

Colors, sounds, shapes, air quality, furniture arrangements, and many more environmental factors have a powerful effect on how you and every member of your team feel when at work. These feelings affect your energy and ability to focus not only on tasks, but on customers.

The sad thing is that, typically, work teams resign themselves to their work spaces. They treat them as givens or facts of life, not as variables that they can alter in order to foster more positive feelings— feelings that make it easier and more comfortable to do their demanding work.

Engage staff in a more proactive approach to their work space. Help them think of ways to become architects who create a space conducive to providing service.

 ### It's Our Place

This tool helps staff to develop a shared vision of a nurturing work space and use that vision to develop quick-fix improvements.[1]

Method

1. Begin by discussing the importance of the environment for customers and staff.

2. Share facts about how colors, smells, sounds, space, light, and other factors can affect people's moods, work habits, and feelings about work.

3. Get people talking about negative and positive environments they've worked in before and the effects these places had on them.

4. Tell the team that you want our place to be the best it can be—to be a place conducive to feeling good about work and serving customers.

5. Introduce a closed-eye process in which you ask them to imagine our space as you would like it to be.

6. Ask the group to close their eyes and try to relax their bodies and forget that they are in a staff meeting. Put on quiet, soothing music and ask people to listen to the music and stop thinking about paperwork, patients, and stress. Ask them to try to relax. Visualization techniques can help. Here are some samples:

Sample Script for Visualization

- Imagine you're waking up on a beautiful sunny day and you feel wonderful. Imagine getting ready for work, but on this day, there is no pressure, no hurry. You are very relaxed and looking forward to the day.
- Imagine coming to work still feeling very peaceful and clear. Absorb the sounds and sights. What do you see and hear as you come to work today, in your ideal fantasy?
- You are walking into our area now, and it's just the way you always wanted it to be. What are you seeing around you? What is your first impression?

7. Continue this way for five minutes, asking them to imagine colors, arrangement of furniture, and so on. Take them on a tour of your entire work area, one part at a time. At each spot, stop and ask, "What are you seeing? What looks different in your ideal?" Also, ask about the sounds or smells they might be experiencing. Ask them how staff and customers seem in this new environment.

8. After 5 to 10 minutes, ask people to get into small groups (2 to 6 people) and share their impressions, listening for common themes.

9. Have small groups present their themes to the whole group.

10. Engage the group in drawing conclusions. Ask these questions:
    —What can we do right now to reach our ideal?
    —What longer-term projects are possible and affordable and will help us approach our ideal?

Variations

- Instead of having teams merely report their findings to the whole group, ask them first to share what they have in common in small teams and then to draw pictures of the ideal space. This makes the activity more fun but does take more time.
- Instead of using the guided visualization technique, ask people to imagine their work space as a garden. Pass out paper and pens and ask them to draw the ideal garden and to embellish this with descriptive words. After individuals do this, ask them to share their images with the whole group. Then, together, look for common themes and ways to institute immediate improvements.

Tips

- Because this activity focuses staff on what they can do and control, it's especially useful if staff have been complaining about the work space, because it helps them focus on aspects other than size. It's also helpful if they've expressed envy or resentment about other people's spaces that have undergone renovation.
- Don't take shortcuts when introducing this activity. Help staff discuss fully how the space affects people's feelings. Encourage them to talk about what they like and don't like at home and in other places.

Space Audit

This tool helps staff examine their work space closely, identify its effects, and generate doable changes they can make to create a space more conducive to serving customers and feeling good about their service.

Method

1. Set up a space team consisting of a few people in your service who want to look at the physical space through the eyes of customers.

2. Arrange for them to walk through every nook and cranny of your space (for example, closets, reception area, exam rooms, testing spaces, lounges, and so on) and address these questions as they go from area to area:

   —What do you hear? How quiet is the space? What effect do the sounds have on you?

   —What do you smell? What are the effects of the smells?

   —What is the quality of light? Is it harsh or soothing? Does it encourage peaceful feelings?

   —What are people allowed to see? What are the effects?

   —What is the level of cleanliness?

   —Does what you see, hear, smell, and feel enhance or detract from the patient/family experience? The staff experience? How?

   —What signs say "No . . . it's not our policy"?

   —Is there any unnecessary clutter?

   —Identify pockets of space that are nurturing.

   —What about areas where staff lounge, if any? Are there fliers on the walls? Is it clean? Uncluttered? Peaceful? Is it a place to rest or keep on working? What is the noise level? The lighting? And what are the effects of all of this?

3. Ask the space team to write up their findings into four categories: see, hear, smell, and feel, as shown in the following example.

See	Hear	Smell	Feel
clutter	people yelling	rotten food on desk	stress from staff
backs of computers	files banging	oil smell	tense
handwritten, torn sign	two radios on different stations		distracted

4. Then, set up a 30-minute space audit feedback session with all staff.

   —Beforehand, ask the space team to prepare to present their findings to staff, using a flipchart to display key points.

   —For the first 10 minutes, ask the space team to report their findings to staff, using their flipcharts to guide them.

—For the next 10 minutes, divide into four small groups, one for "see," one for "hear," one for "smell," and one for "feel." If you have more than 16 people, have duplicate groups for each sense, so that there aren't more than four people per group. Have individuals from the space team facilitate each small group. Have each group do the following:

–Brainstorm ideas for changing the space related to the category they were assigned.

–Prioritize their five favorite ideas.

—During the last 10 minutes, do the following activities:

–Invite the groups to present their priority ideas to the large group and encourage discussion.

–Sort out the ideas into those that are clearly workable, unworkable, and possible but have to be placed on hold.

–Before leaving, invite staff to become involved in making the changes identified as workable. Consider having the space team coordinate implementation of ideas or divide into miniteams of two or three, each agreeing to implement one of the ideas. Ask the teams to create a plan, set a deadline, and check back with you regularly.

Variation

• Instead of dividing up by sense, divide into miniteams with each team responsible for one section of your work space (for example, one miniteam responsible for the exam room, one for the reception area, and so on). Your goal is to have the sum total of all teams work to complete this chart and then develop ideas in response to their findings.

	Waiting Area	Staff Lounge	Exam Room	Work Area
See				
Hear				
Smell				
Feel				

Tips

- Implement this quickly. The space audit, staff meeting, and completion of initial changes should take no more than a month for the easy-to-fix space glitches. You and your staff should be able to see, hear, smell, and feel differences within a month if you want people to feel encouraged by the immediacy of a more conducive work space.
- Be sure to tell your staff up front what will not work. Tell them the constraints. Otherwise, they might build false hopes and end up disillusioned and disappointed. If they can't relocate walls, for instance, tell them so up front.

Summary of Approach 1

In approach 1, you focused on helping people create a more conducive physical environment for service delivery—a nurturing environment for themselves. Although the physical environment doesn't affect some people's feelings all that much, others are affected. Changes your team makes to create a more comfortable environment will soothe nerves day in and day out. That's what makes the time expenditure worthwhile.

Approach 2: Personal Coping Skills in a High-Stress Environment

The environment is one variable that affects people's feelings and energy. The next question is, How can you help staff develop the personal coping skills they sorely need when working in a high-stress environment? That's not environmental; that's internal!

The secret: Help staff take better care of themselves during times of stress. Help them take responsibility for learning ways to cope with and manage first their own stress and then other people's stress.

The fact is, things happen that trigger stress. By and large, people can't prevent many of the stressful things that happen. But, they can learn to manage their response to these situations, so that they are not debilitated, drained, or otherwise hampered. In service environments, people benefit greatly from being able to contain and control their own responses to stressful situations. At the same time, they need to know how to best handle other people, specifically stressed-out coworkers whose negativity, if left to its own devices, becomes contagious for the rest of the team.

This next section presents many effective tools. Consider devoting a few minutes of a weekly staff meeting to acknowledging the stress people are under and presenting one tool a week (or have a respected colleague present it).

 ### Relaxation Exercises

How often have people told you and your staff to just relax? The question is *how?* Teach your staff these techniques one at a time to help them know how they can take a breather or calm themselves down on the job. The following tools are excerpted from *Stress Management for Professionals in Health Care* by Wendy Leebov (Beaverton, OR: Mosby Great Performance, 1996, pp. 34–36). Each of these tools can be done in less than five minutes.

Five-Step Relaxation
This exercise relaxes your body, leaves your mind free to work on the problems you are facing, and generates the calm energy you need to accomplish difficult tasks:

1. Find a comfortable place to sit.
2. Place your feet flat on the floor.
3. Close your eyes.
4. Breathe steadily with purpose for about five minutes.
5. Pay close attention to the parts of your body that feel tense and will them to relax.

Progressive Relaxation
This exercise helps your team learn to relax by tightening up! Experts have developed a very effective technique for muscle relaxation that leaves you feeling relaxed and refreshed.

1. One muscle group at a time, tense up. For instance, tense up your eye muscles, then your cheek muscles, then your neck muscles, then your shoulder muscles, and so on. Concentrating on one muscle group at a time, hold the tension for five seconds and then release it slowly while silently saying to yourself, "Relax and let go."

2. Take a deep breath.
3. As you breathe out slowly, silently say to yourself, "Relax and let go."
4. Follow this process for each part of your body. For instance, when focusing on your neck do the following:
   —Push your head back, tense up, and relax according to the instructions.
   —Bring your head forward to touch your chest and do the same.
   —Roll your head to your right shoulder and then to your left shoulder.
5. Repeat the same process for your head, shoulders, arms and hands, chest and lungs, back, abdomen, hips, and legs and feet.

Deep Breathing

Deep breathing facilitates relaxation in an atmosphere of stress, worry, or pressure.

1. Inhale deeply through your nose.
2. Feel your stomach expand as you inhale so that you fill your lungs completely.
3. Let the air out slowly through your mouth. Exhale completely. As you let the air out, your stomach should contract.
4. Relax and then repeat.

Breathing to a Count

1. Inhale slowly through your nose while counting to three.
2. Exhale slowly while counting to three.
3. Count to three again and tell yourself to relax.
4. Repeat this sequence for about two minutes and you will feel the tension drain from your body.

Scanning Relaxation

With scanning relaxation, you use your inner awareness, not your eyes, to scan your body in order to pinpoint any areas of tension:

1. Inhale while scanning one area of your body for tension. As you breathe out, relax that area.
2. Proceed through each area of your body, scanning it for tension and relaxing each part. Include your face and neck, your

shoulders and arms, your chest and lungs, your abdomen, your hips, and your legs and feet.

Imagery

Most people struggle with unwelcome thoughts about a difficult problem at work or problems in their personal lives. One thought leads to another, and you end up feeling worked up and frazzled, as though your head were spinning. Imagery techniques replace your distressed thinking with calming images. This stops your mind from racing wildly, and after relaxing, you gain new perspective on the problem.

1. Imagine a pleasant scene: While concentrating in a quiet place, allow yourself to daydream, creating a very relaxing, pleasant scene or re-creating a place that you have seen many times.
2. Picture it in your mind's eye. Try to relive your experience there mentally in every way you possibly can, remembering both sights and sounds.
3. Later, when you're nervous or distressed, take a few minutes to visit that place in your mind, replaying your pleasant experience there. This has a calming effect.

Instead of retreating to their own pleasant scene, some people listen to a tape or respond as a friend reads a guided imagery exercise to them. For example, picture yourself walking along a warm, sunny beach along the edge of crystal-clear blue water. You hear the waves rush. . . . You feel the warm, clean sand between your toes. . . . You smell the fresh salt air.

Tips

- Staff can do these relaxation methods on the run. Encourage staff to equip themselves with these self-control devices to take the edge off the anxiety-producing or exhausting aspects of their service to customers.
- The one-tool-a-week approach helps people develop this relaxation tool kit.

It's Your Time Out

This tool will help your staff identify healthy versus unhealthy ways to spend precious time-outs during the workday.[2]

Method

1. Begin by discussing the importance of time-outs during the day as an opportunity to reenergize, regroup, recoup, and reconnect. These time-outs may be official or unofficial breaks, depending on your team, the work you're doing, union regulations, and so on. The point is, there are healthy and less healthy ways to spend downtime.
2. Brainstorm with the group examples of healthy and productive versus unhealthy, unproductive ways to spend time-outs.

Positive Ways to Spend Time-Outs	Negative Ways to Spend Time-Outs
•	•
•	•
•	•
•	•

3. Ask the group to look over the list and identify ways they spend time-outs most often. Ask, "Are these the most helpful, nurturing ways for you to spend your time-outs? What could you be doing instead?"

Tips

- This activity raises awareness about what staff are already doing. Since it's not easy to get some staff to take responsibility for taking care of themselves, this activity works best when viewed by staff as one of the many things we can do to take care of ourselves.

- If staff feel that they are being judged, they will clam up. Be careful to sound supportive, not judgmental.

Know Thyself

Help staff identify their own responses to unpleasant experiences with customers and coworkers, examine the effectiveness of these responses, and consider alternative ways to handle themselves more effectively with this tool.[3]

Method

1. Introduce the idea that most people have patterns of response to unpleasant experiences with customers and coworkers.
2. Ask people to complete the "What Do *You* Do?" worksheet.

What Do You Do?

Think about the following list and check off things you do when you've had a particularly unpleasant experience with a customer or coworker. Do you . . .		
	Yes	No
Let off steam with the next available person?		
Go off to a quiet place to calm down and get yourself together?		
Push it aside and go on with your work?		
Talk about the other person and what they did to upset you?		
Find someone who has it just as bad, or worse, and commiserate?		
Find someone to talk it out with in the hopes of calming down and eventually working it out?		
Look for something pleasant to do to switch your focus temporarily?		

Other responses:

In what ways do the ones you checked work for you?

In what ways do the ones you checked not work for you?

What are some things that might work instead?

3. Ask them to share their results in groups of three and get advice from their group mates on the last question.

Tips

- Help staff compare their best techniques and also commit themselves to replacing one dysfunctional technique with a better one.
- To make it safer to talk about these, give examples that are true for you.

We're Only Human!

This tool relieves pressure on staff by giving them permission to have negative feelings about customers and coworkers, recognize these, and still behave appropriately.

Method

1. In a staff meeting, introduce the topic of considering the feelings they carry around with them all day, some of which are negative toward customers and coworkers. Make these points:
   —Such feelings are, of course, normal. Everyone has some. And it doesn't mean that you're an unfeeling caregiver when you harbor such feelings.

—There are many times when customers push our buttons and
we can't say what we want to say because, after all, they are
the customers! Today is an opportunity to look at how to
handle these situations.

2. Divide people into small groups (for example, three or four)
and give each group a piece of flipchart paper. Ask one person
per group to serve as recorder.

3. Have the small groups list everything they ever wanted to say to
a customer, but couldn't. Give people 10 minutes.

4. When finished, convene everyone and ask one person per group
at a time to stand and say three things from their lists. Go from
group to group until every group has had a turn.

5. Afterward, ask and record answers on flipcharts:
—How did this feel?
—How many of you suspect that your customers know you feel
that way about them?
—How would they know (for example, tone of voice, facial
expressions, and so on)?

6. Ask the group to swap the helpful and unhelpful things they
can do with these feelings (for example, talk to a friend, exercise, breathe deeply, set limits, go to a quiet place to relax for a
few minutes).

7. Close the discussion by emphasizing the need to express feelings
in a constructive way, because bottled-up or ignored feelings
tend to leak out in unconstructive ways.

 Tips

• Do this in a spirit of technique swapping. This is not therapy
after all, nor are the techniques that will be discussed the be-all
and end-all of coping with negative feelings.

• Let your team know that you support their using each other to
vent frustrations and negative feelings, pointing out that the listener needs to be objective and careful not to join a downward
spiral of cynicism. Refer to a future staff meeting discussion
about how to be on the receiving end with a colleague, listening
in a way that does not drag you, the listener, down.

Dealing with Negativity

The above tools help staff identify dysfunctional patterns that take their toll on people operating in a stressful atmosphere. This next section focuses on how to deal with the negativity that surrounds you, so that it doesn't drag you down.

Negativity drains people's energy from service delivery. People too often get caught up in another person's negativity. Most work groups have one or two people who are the naysayers, the complainers, the exhausted ones, or the cynics. While you need to address the effects of their attitudes on service performance, make sure that you also stop their feelings from being contagious. Negative feelings are compelling and attract other staff's attention, and responding to the negative people consumes the precious energy of people who feel differently.

Help your staff develop individual tools and a sense of responsibility that enables them to resist the contagion of negative, cynical feelings among coworkers. You'll stem the tide of negativity and see better, more energetic service to customers as a result.

Present these next tools in a series called I Don't Need to Get Caught. These tools help individuals avoid joining in with or absorbing a colleague's negativity or frustration.

The Vicious Cycle

This tool has three purposes:

1. To help staff recognize that the feelings they have about their work and customers affect their actions and behaviors—and that these actions and behaviors affect their outcomes and results
2. To help staff identify chain reactions they experience at work
3. To help them learn to continue positive chain reactions and stop negative chain reactions in their tracks

Method
1. Pass out the handout titled "The Vicious Cycle."

The Vicious Cycle

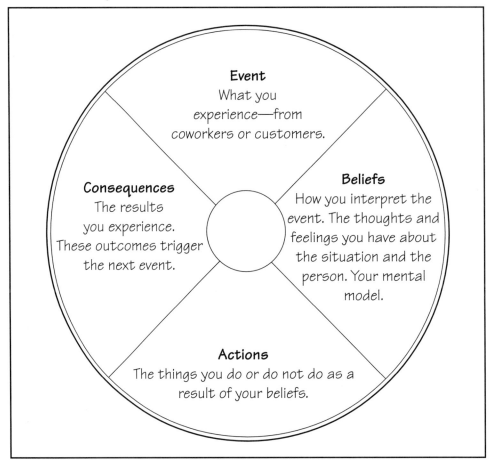

Event
What you experience—from coworkers or customers.

Beliefs
How you interpret the event. The thoughts and feelings you have about the situation and the person. Your mental model.

Actions
The things you do or do not do as a result of your beliefs.

Consequences
The results you experience. These outcomes trigger the next event.

Reprinted, with permission, from Gail Scott & Associates © 1997

2. Explain the four points in the cycle to help staff see that their interpretations of people and situations greatly influence the things they do.

3. Use the events identified on the "What Do *You* Do?" handout to make your points. Emphasize that when people are interpreting actions and words of other people, they have choices. They can make certain assumptions that will lead to one set of behaviors, or they can choose to interpret the individual or situation differently and as a result behave quite differently.

What Do You Do?

Events	Beliefs: Why It Pushes Your Buttons	Actions: What You Would Like to Say or Do	Actions: What You Could Say or Do Instead (if you interpret the behavior differently)
Threats: "If you don't get this fixed right away, I'll speak to _____."	Assumes that you broke it, did it on purpose, and can fix it by yourself.	Tell the person where they can go.	
Sarcasm: "You really look like you're in a big rush to take care of it. Ha-ha!"	Assumes you wouldn't like to take care of it right away.	Explain all the other priorities you have and that this just isn't high on the list.	
Insinuations: "I already told you how to do this. Don't we have any competent people here?"	Assumes you don't know what you are doing.	Want to say: "If you explained it so someone could understand it, then there wouldn't be a problem."	
Other:			
Other:			

Reprinted, with permission, from Gail Scott & Associates © 1997

4. After you discuss the three sample situations, break the group into smaller groups of three and ask them to generate real cases from their experience. Give the groups several minutes and have them share the results with everyone. Encourage them to talk about why their interpretations push their buttons and set off the vicious cycle.

5. Ask them to discuss situations that are particularly difficult, particularly easy, and any lessons they received from this exercise.

Tips

• Have people work in small groups, so that they can help each other see the extent to which they fall into the vicious cycle and talk each other out of it. Other people can help to shift one's perspective.

- People can have big breakthroughs when they realize that they probably cannot change others' (for example, customers') behavior, but they can indeed alter their own responses to those behaviors and produce better outcomes for both the customers and themselves.

 ## Five Steps to Keeping Your Cool under Pressure

This tool goes a step beyond the vicious cycle discussion by helping staff develop alternative ways keeping their calm. Its purpose is to help staff develop a tool kit of ways to maintain or regain composure when they find themselves on the receiving end of stress and pressure.

Method

1. Distribute the "Five Steps to Help You Keep Your Cool" and "Keeping Your Cool" techniques.

Five Steps to Help You Keep Your Cool

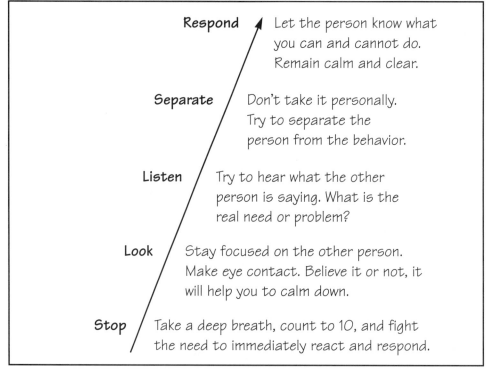

Respond — Let the person know what you can and cannot do. Remain calm and clear.

Separate — Don't take it personally. Try to separate the person from the behavior.

Listen — Try to hear what the other person is saying. What is the real need or problem?

Look — Stay focused on the other person. Make eye contact. Believe it or not, it will help you to calm down.

Stop — Take a deep breath, count to 10, and fight the need to immediately react and respond.

Reprinted, with permission, from Gail Scott & Associates © 1997

Keeping Your Cool Techniques

Technique	How It Works
Stop	Let the other person blow off steam—until they "hit the wall." Nod empathetically. Don't fight back or respond to their accusations or threats. This works initially because you are not adding any negative energy to the situation or giving the other person anything to respond to.
Look	Stay focused on the other person. Making eye contact says that you are listening to them. It works because the individual wants to be heard.
Listen	Identify the underlying feeling (anger, frustration, disappointment, fear) and affirm your understanding. (For example, "I can appreciate how you feel in this situation.") This works because it helps to diffuse the anger. Hopefully, it will calm the person down.
Separate	Don't get caught up in the behavior. Stay focused on the problem. Affirm your commitment to find a workable solution. (For example, "I would like to be able to work something out. Let me see how I can help.")
Respond	Let the person know what you can do. Set limits if necessary. Let the other person know what is and isn't acceptable, while affirming your desire to help. (For example, "I really want to help, but I can't if you continue to _____. I think we could work this out a lot better if we _____.")

2. Review the five steps using specific examples (your own or those included on the "Sticky Situations" sheet).

Sticky Situations

Situation	Get Yourself Together	Separate the Person from the Problem	Hear What the Person Has to Say	Respond with Limits and "Can-Dos"
Doctor says you don't know what you are doing because s/he hasn't received information s/he expected. Actually, s/he didn't request the material in a way that others understood.				
Patient's family blames you for not taking patient to see therapist. Actually, the patient refused to go.				
Coworker accuses you and others of misplacing patient-related file. Actually, you had nothing to do with it but have some ideas for improving the filing system.				
Patient accuses you of not giving the right treatment. Actually, you followed orders but do have some questions regarding the treatment.				

3. Divide the group into threes and distribute the "Sticky Situation" handout. Ask the groups to designate each member as person A, B, or C.

—For the first round, A's play the upset person and B's try to apply the five steps in response. The C's observe to see what worked and what didn't and then give feedback.

—Rotate roles and let the B's have a shot at keeping their cool. Continue again with C's.

4. Ask the group to discuss what was easy, hard, and any lessons from the experience.

5. If time permits, continue with real situations.

Tips

- As you review the five techniques, ask the group to draw from their experiences to explain why each works. It's important that those few people in the group who believe that nothing will ever work hear people describe times these techniques have worked for them.

- The fact is, there are some people whom you cannot win over, no matter what you do. The respond technique involves setting limits with the other person, which in many cases is all you can do. Its effect is to help you keep your calm.

- Deepen people's thinking by asking them to cite worst-case scenarios or situations when each technique will not work. Then, ask them why they think it did not work. For instance, some think that if a customer continues to yell and threatens to speak to your supervisor, the technique didn't work. The fact is, it didn't work only if the employee lost her cool. Emphasize that you can't always calm down the other person, but you can learn to avoid getting caught up in other people's anger. If we can remain calm, set limits, and state calmly what we can and cannot do, then we have succeeded. Not every situation can be turned into a win-win situation.

Approach 3: Build a Supportive Work Team

So far, we shared ways staff can take care of themselves under pressure, either by removing themselves from stressful situations, doing relaxation exercises, learning ways to respond differently when they feel attacked, and learning to keep their cool. Since there are changes and people who inevitably make work difficult, these techniques will hopefully help staff cope more effectively.

Another approach that we do have control over if we choose to exercise it is how we treat each other. A supportive work team can go far to help staff manage under pressure and deal effectively with difficult people and situations. The reverse is also true. A team that does not work well together and support each other makes matters much worse, and that's the last thing customers and staff need.

Begin working with staff to develop a shared vision of a supportive work team and then help staff translate this vision into reality. Use the tools offered here in staff meetings. Each one can be completed within an hour, or combine several to use as a plan for a longer staff retreat focused on the goal of developing a team that works together to provide excellent service to customers.

Imagining the Ideal

Help staff create a vision of a supportive work team and then translate this vision into actions and behaviors with this creative tool.[4]

Method

1. Ask the group to form pairs. Have pairs interview each other on their experience or involvement in a team that they felt was extremely supportive. After a few minutes, ask partners to share their experiences with the whole group. Capture the common themes on a whiteboard or flipchart page. As people call out themes, ask, "What about this attribute created a feeling of support within the team?" You will probably hear responses such as respecting each other's viewpoints, being direct and honest with each other, listening to each other, helping each other with tasks, and sharing knowledge and information. As the group is sharing, feel free to add qualities that you also think are important.

2. Once you have a substantial list, look for ways to combine or group similar attributes. You're likely to end up with from five to eight characteristics of a supportive work team.

3. Divide the group into as many subgroups as there are characteristics. Give each group a flipchart page and a marker. Ask groups to spend 10 minutes further defining the characteristics, thinking them through, and generating specific examples and ways they can demonstrate the characteristic.

4. The small groups then share their lists with everyone and invite questions and additional examples.

5. Ask for volunteers to work on refining the lists, eliminating overlap, and editing to achieve consistent, clear language. Or

send the raw material out to everyone and invite people to suggest refinements to submit to you before the next meeting.

6. Conclude the meeting by holding a discussion about the kinds of behaviors that are not supportive (for example, talking behind each other's back, and so on). Push for specifics and fine points. Invite controversy, because sometimes people's ideas about support are not well thought out. For instance, some staff will say that having a shoulder to cry on is supportive. But not necessarily. Sometimes, it isn't. The person may actually need help reframing a situation or a nudge to change his own approach, instead of getting endless sympathy and encouragement to keep feeling upset. Also, some say that pitching in and lending a hand is supportive, but not always. When someone is trying to learn something and someone else pitches in, they may prevent the person from having the experience she needs. Leave time here for substantive, thought-provoking discussion.

7. Explain that this activity is the first step in developing coworker norms related to having a supportive work team. Ask people to think further about ways the group is and isn't supportive of each other.

Tips

- This activity can generate discomfort if the group is having difficulties with one another in their everyday work. Start with a discussion of the benefits of having a supportive work team for them as individuals, for the group, and for customers.

- Don't eliminate the discussion of what does *not* constitute support. Talk about how support has changed over the years. Invite people to share views about the relationship between support and dependence.

Building Partners for Support

The first step in building a supportive work team involves fleshing out the characteristics; the second challenge is making them operational. This tool helps you develop partners for success by using peer coaches and mentors.[5]

Method

1. Ask the group to consider the qualities of an effective and an ineffective coach.
   —Start with an effective coach: Look for suggestions such as "Brings out the best in people, helps them achieve their goals, provides guidance," and so on.
   —Ask the group to identify behaviors that an effective coach avoids, such as doing the job for people, instead of helping them do it themselves.
2. Pass out the six-step coaching model and walk through it.

Six-Step Peer Coaching Model

Step 1: Ask the person to describe the situation.

Step 2: Ask, "What about the situation bothered you?"

Step 3: Ask, "What would you have liked to have happened in this situation?"

Step 4: Ask, "What did you do and what did the other person do that contributed to the negative outcome?"

Step 5: Ask, "Is there anything you see now that you could have done differently?"

Step 6: Ask, "What do you think could help you in the future?"

3. Tell the group that they will engage in an activity designed to help them to help each other in sticky situations with customers. The twist is that they will be asked to coach and support each other, yet not intervene or take over the situation with the customer.
4. Divide the group into trios and have them decide who is person A, B, and C in their group. A is the coach, B is the person being coached, and C is the observer.
   —B thinks of a recent situation with a customer that didn't have a positive result. (For some reason, the customer was difficult or the situation was sticky.)
   —Ask A to follow the six-step peer coaching model to help B and C think through the process and pinpoint how they felt, when they got hooked, what happened, and what they could have done differently.

—At the end of this brief discussion, ask C to give feedback to both parties, pointing out what he saw as effective and offering suggestions for greater effectiveness. A and B can also give feedback to each other.

—Repeat the process, rotating roles so that all three people in the trio have a turn as coach, coached, and observer.

5. Reconvene the whole group and ask what made the experience hard and easy, and invite lessons.

6. Ask the trios to use the coaching model with each other during the week to capture further learning for the group.

Variation

• Some people get frustrated if their partner doesn't offer suggestions. Consider making step 5 in the model a brainstorm of all present possible alternatives; in step 6 the person clarifies which ideas and suggestions are most useful or applicable.

Tips

• Good groups will catch on to this model quickly. Still, spend a few minutes setting norms and warming up so people will be self-disclosing with each other.

• Make sure everyone gets a turn. Otherwise, only those who had a chance to try out the coach role will realize how easy and helpful it is to follow this model.

Conclusion

These are tough times. You can't remove all sources of stress on staff, and you can't effectively take responsibility for cushioning people against the stresses they feel. The best you can do is to help them help themselves. Help them work together to create a more conducive and comfortable physical work space. Help them develop personal coping skills so that they can manage their personal responses to stress and also avoid getting depleted by the stresses others feel. You can help your team develop norms that foster mutual support for serving customers well in the face of uncomfortable stress.

All of this takes time and attention at a cost to the organization. But the costs to the organization of *not* building staff resilience, positivism, and mutual support are much greater.

Notes

1. Adapted, with permission, from Gail Scott and Associates © 1997.

2. Ibid.

3. Ibid.

4. Ibid.

5. Ibid.

Chapter 7

• • •

Maintain Your Focus
on Service

Do You Need to Read This Chapter?

Eavesdrop for a minute. We interviewed managers who have been involved in service improvement for a long time and asked, "What's hard about maintaining your service focus over the long haul?" This is what they had to say:

- During the minutes and hours when we're actually doing service-related work, things go better. But then, we move on to other things and service slips. It's as if there are compartments in our minds. When we're in the service compartment, we're service oriented and we make good decisions for our customers. But then, we leave the service compartment and enter another one, like the financial compartment or the "what about me?" compartment, and we seem to forget totally about service. That's when we get in trouble and do things that work against our service commitment.
- With so many priorities competing for staff time and attention and so much work to do, people's stamina for working on service fades. There's just too much to do—too much to keep in mind. They get overwhelmed by it all. They complain that they can't work on everything at once! And they're right! So, what can I say?
- My staff are human. As hard as they work, they need and expect to feel appreciated for how hard they work and for their

dedication to customers. But the minute we solve one service problem, we speed on to the next one, forgetting to stop and appreciate what we've accomplished. And what happens? Staff think, "After all I've done, who knows and who cares!" They feel unappreciated and that kills morale. People turn into martyrs instead of feeling proud and effective. And their martyrdom doesn't do much for the atmosphere. People run out of steam and don't want to keep up the good work.

These words convey the frustrations many managers experience as they try to maintain their service focus over the long run. If you share any of these concerns, read on. In this chapter we introduce and explain three ways to give your service focus staying power and offer options for accomplishing each one. Here they are in a nutshell:

1. Mainstream your service focus: Integrate it into everyday activities and routines.
2. Stop overwhelming people with too many service priorities: Focus on service improvement one behavior at a time.
3. Stop speeding on to the next problem before you appreciate progress already made: Recognize people for their hard work and results when customers are happier and service is improving.

Mainstream Your Service Focus

Imagine this relationship situation between two loved ones. They experience problems with each other. One perceives the other as inconsiderate or withholding in his or her communication and asserts that this is hurting their relationship. The other is concerned about this and suggests going to family counseling. The two go to counseling and discuss their communication. In the process, the counselor suggests several approaches that will improve the couple's communication, including listening, reflecting back what they heard, and responding to feelings. Both parties agree to try these and, in the sessions, they practice. In fact, they do a wonderful job of communicating openly and responding to each other's feelings. But then, in between sessions, they fall back into their old patterns and their distance from one another returns. This goes on, with steps forward during counseling and steps backward upon returning home. Both parties realize that they are capable of great communication because they show this during the sessions; but then it stops there, and home is no happier than it was. In fact, some resentment even builds over time. The challenge here is how to internalize the new skills so that they pop up at home and everywhere, not just in the counselor's office.

The dynamic is similar with a service focus. Some teams do dynamite things and make dynamite decisions when they're explicitly focusing on service improvement. But then the pressures of everyday work return, and their service focus simmers on a back burner instead of providing energy and direction for the challenge at hand.

The challenge then is how to infuse everything you and your team do with your service focus. How can you take it out of the compartment and make it pervasive, so you make those sparks of progress ignite every facet of your team's work?

In this section, we present four tools that will help you bring your service focus out of the compartment and into the air that your staff breathes. Briefly, these are the tools:

- Do a "missed opportunities" audit to identify compartments that your service focus has not entered—and open the door.
- Use a meeting screen that pushes you to take your service focus to meetings with you.
- Use quick service warm-ups at staff meetings to keep staff eyes on service.
- Apply and promote a service lens in discussions with your team and the individuals on it.

Missed Opportunities Audit

This tool is diagnostic. It helps you identify those compartments or aspects of your service in which your service focus is alive and well versus those compartments that are as yet untouched by your service commitment. Once you diagnose these areas, you are in a better position to do what's needed to apply your service focus there, too. Note also that this tool helps you identify gaps you can fill by reading other chapters of this book.

Method

1. At a staff meeting, announce the purposes of the missed opportunities audit. Ask for volunteers. They'll need to complete a short survey and then attend a meeting where everyone who completed the questionnaire discusses the results and develops remedies.
2. Tailor this survey to your needs by adding questions suited to your service and omitting those that don't apply.

Missed Opportunities Audit

Circle 1 for Hardly; 2 for Somewhat, and 3 for Quite a bit

If someone sat in on our meetings, how visible would our service commitment be?   1   2   3

If someone looked at our budget decisions, how much would our commitment to customer service show?   1   2   3

If someone looked at our job descriptions, how clear would it be that we're committed to impressive customer service?   1   2   3

If a group of consumers walked into our service and scrutinized the physical environment, how clear would it be to them that we're committed to customer comfort and satisfaction?   1   2   3

How well does the form we use for staff performance appraisal reflect our commitment to service and customer satisfaction?   1   2   3

When we look at all the things that get measured in our service, how visible is our concern for customer satisfaction?   1   2   3

(If your service has a board) How much do reports to our board and meetings with them highlight our service focus versus focusing on other things?   1   2   3

If we listed all the committees and task forces that staff participate on, to what extent does the lion's share lead ultimately to a positive impact on customers?   1   2   3

Think about all the ways members of our team now
get recognized and appreciated. To what extent do
we appreciate and recognize people for contributions
to impressive service and satisfying customers?   1   2   3

Look at all the printed material that can be seen by
customers and also everything we mail out to customers. To what extent does our commitment to
customer satisfaction show in the printed material
posted in-house and sent out?   1   2   3

When people get hired for this service, how much attention goes to ensuring that their interaction style and
demeanor will be satisfying to our customers?   1   2   3

When new staff come on board, how much attention
do we give to service expectations in their initial
orientation?   1   2   3

When service breaks down because of individuals on
the team behaving inappropriately, how likely is it
that someone on the team will confront them on
their behavior and its effects on customers?   1   2   3

[Add your own questions here]   1   2   3

3. After your committee members fill this out individually, convene
   them and tally the numbers in response to each item. Then, on a
   flipchart, list the items, starting with those with the lowest scores.
   These reflect the compartments in your service that have been left
   relatively untouched by your service commitment.
4. For each of the top five, discuss possible remedies—actions
   people can take to raise the score by injecting your service
   commitment somehow into that compartment. For each, see if
   there is a doable approach and decide how you can collectively
   get this done using existing resources. Use a format like the
   following:

If This Is True	Consider This
If your service focus is relatively absent from meetings	• Try tool 2 below, the meeting screen • In chapter 2, consult the tool called Mike Ustomer • Create a customer hat and ask one staff member per meeting to wear it and listen/observe from the point of view of the customer, intervening when the customer perspective is missing or skewed.
If your budget decisions don't reflect your commitment to customer service	• Use the current budget for practice. Convene a committee to examine how decisions might have differed if your customers' top-priority needs had been dominant during decision making. • Look at the current budget and ask what trade-offs or changes you can make to put this year's money where your rhetoric is about satisfying your customers' top-priority needs from both your services and your staff. • When developing next year's budget, consider assigning to the team a staff member to serve as the team's customer service watchdog, who questions decisions and their impact from a customer service perspective.
If job descriptions don't show your service focus	• Insert the same line in everyone's job description, such as, "Makes decisions and behaves in ways that reflect impressive service to both internal and external customers." • Spell out in every job description the particular role this position has in fostering excellent customer service. For instance, "The receptionist identifies self and greets people in person and on the phone quickly and in a professional and friendly manner, so that customers are immediately impressed."

If your physical environment doesn't show your commitment to customer comfort and satisfaction	• Invite in consumer to audit your environment and make very specific suggestions. • Form a staff committee to do a customer focus group (see chapter 3 of this book) on your service's environment and then initiate an agenda of improvements.
If your performance appraisal forms don't reflect your commitment to service and customer satisfaction	• Add to these forms whatever customer-oriented behavior statements you have or that you added to staff job descriptions.
If service and customer satisfaction aren't measured much or well	• Read chapter 3 on how to institute methods of listening in to the voices of your customers. • Invite satisfaction measurement vendors to educate you about what's involved in satisfaction surveys. Then, either purchase the best service you can find and afford; or, if you're penniless or have internal measurement experts, develop your own.
If reports to your board don't show your service focus	• Change your report formats. Develop a balanced scorecard that shows both financial information, quality information, and customer satisfaction indicators. • Work with the appropriate board members or committee of the board to alter the format of the information they want from you. Suggest a standing committee report on service quality and customer satisfaction.
If most committees and task forces that consume staff time fail to lead ultimately to a positive impact on customers	• Pretend you have no committees or task forces. Make people justify any that they think are needed, with customer impact as a component of the justification. Starting from zero, restore only those committees that can justify the time consumed by impact on customers or other compelling results. • Abolish all committees and task forces that don't have a phenomenal justification, because they eat up time that could otherwise be spent on serving and satisfying customers.

If your recognition practices don't focus enough on contributors to impressing customers	• Form a short-term committee to do the following: —Examine the options presented in part 3 of this chapter and decide on an efficient mix of methods that will focus people on service accomplishments and people who satisfy customers. —Abolish recognition practices that don't have positive effects, so you replace wasted efforts with effective methods.
If printed material doesn't highlight your focus on pleasing customers	• Collect all of your written materials. Hold a focus group of former customers and invite their feedback about these printed materials. • Develop a team to rewrite/change the materials to better meet customer needs and reflect your customer focus. Invite customer feedback once again before the revisions go to print.
If you don't screen job candidates for service effectiveness If the way you orient new staff doesn't pay much attention to service expectations	• Read chapter 2 of this book and follow suit. • Develop a checklist for people who orient new staff. Include these items and do them as part of every new person's orientation: —Did manager sit down with new person and share personal commitment to service quality and express hope and expectation that new person will contribute to the high standards of service here? —Did someone show service expectations, service scripts, and protocols to new person? —Did someone link new person with service star and ask service star to show them the ropes? —Did someone introduce new person to customers and ask customers to tell the new person what's important to them about service and what impresses them?

If people who dissatisfy customers receive little or no feedback	• Read in chapter 1 about resolving mixed feelings. • Embrace your role as coach and talk with staff who violate standards. Stop letting these opportunities pass. Set an example. • At a staff meeting, engage staff in discussing the consequences of holding back feedback when coworkers dissatisfy customers. See if you can agree on a signal or method for giving feedback. • Have a staff meeting on how to give constructive feedback. (See features of helpful feedback in chapter 2.)

5. By identifying these opportunities and making plans, you can spread your service focus throughout your service. People spend gigantic amounts of time in committees, meetings, and retreats. And no doubt, your service is subject to at least dozens and even hundreds of policies and procedures. The challenge is to infuse all of these with your customers' voices. The patients' and customers' needs should be the recurrent theme and the chorus. Staff's service commitment is judged by the degree to which they advance customer satisfaction while also meeting your other objectives.

Tips

- If your organization has a human resource staff, ask their help in revamping job descriptions and the performance appraisal and staff-coaching practices to better support your service focus.
- You might find a lot of repair work to do here. Prioritize and do one thing per month. Or invite pairs of staff to revamp one area and have them report back monthly on progress.

Meeting Screen

If your meetings are devoid of your service focus or just so darn time consuming that they take people away from service to customers, you need this tool. It will help remind you and your team to use precious meeting time to advance your customer focus.

Method

Make multiple copies of these questions and distribute them to everyone in charge of meetings or task forces. Ask them to use these as a guide to planning, conducting, and evaluating their meetings to ensure that these meetings advance your service focus and customer satisfaction pursuits.

Meeting Screen on Customer Focus

When planning a meeting, ask the following:

- Is the purpose going to help customers directly or indirectly? If not, is this meeting really necessary?
- What can I add to this agenda to advance our service focus?
- Is there anything on this agenda that I can remove to shorten the meeting, because time spent in meetings steals people away from their valuable work of serving customers?
- Who really needs to be at the meeting and who is better off staying available to customers during this precious time?

During the meeting, post these questions and refer to them to stay on track:

- Are we losing sight of our customers' needs, concerns, and preferences in this discussion?
- Are we being efficient now, or is this meeting stealing time away from serving customers?

To evaluate a meeting, ask the following:

- How valuable was this meeting in improving our services to customers?
- What resulted from this meeting that will help us better serve our customers?
- How well did we use our time, since wasted time takes us away from serving customers?
- Were there people here whose time was not well spent, such that they could have contributed more by being with customers?

Tips

- If people in charge of meetings conscientiously ask these questions of themselves and their groups several meetings in a row, they will eventually internalize these questions and maintain a customer focus in meetings.
- There's no sense distributing this tool unless you, the manager, use it. Be a role model. Show people its value, and act on the findings to reduce meetings that interfere with service and to enhance meetings so they serve a customer-related purpose.

Quick Service Warm-Ups

This tool offers simple ways to begin meetings that not only keep customer service issues primary, but also give your team a lift as they proceed through their busy days or routines. It helps people focus in on the meeting, get energized, and participate from the start by asking them to share on service-related topics.

Method

1. Introduce a ritual of having a short five-minute warm-up activity at every meeting to help people focus.
2. Use service-related warm-ups that keep people thinking and talking about service. Here are a few examples to get you started. Then you can make up your own. Use one per meeting and then invite other topics or start this same list over again (because people will by then have new answers).
3. Introduce the warm-ups. Say, "As a warm-up, let's start by going around and having everyone complete this sentence. If you can't think of something, it's OK to say 'pass' and then at the end, you can have a turn. So, take a minute and think of what you want to say."
   —Warm-up 1: A compliment I got from a customer this week was _____.
   —Warm-up 2: A service improvement I'm personally working on is _____.
   —Warm-up 3: If I ran this service, an improvement I'd make for the sake of our customers is _____.

—Warm-up 4: A tough service situation that came up for me this week was _____.

—Warm-up 5: If we could hear our customers talking about us, I think we'd hear them say _____.

—Warm-up 6: If our customers had a magic wand to make a change in our service, I bet they would _____.

—Warm-up 7: When it comes to serving my customers, I wish I could get some help getting better at _____.

—Warm-up 8: The funniest thing that happened this week between a customer and me was _____.

—Warm-up 9: A great service interaction I noticed a coworker having was when _____.

—Warm-up 10: A time this week when someone here made it easier for me to provide good service was when

_____.

4. At the end, thank people for sharing.

Tips

• Notice that these warm-ups focus on positive events and feelings. Since warm-ups should take only a few minutes, avoid the negative, since otherwise you'll generate problems that you don't have time to address in a thorough and supportive manner.

• Post the warm-up on a chalkboard or flipchart page, so people remember it as you go around.

• Give people a minute to think about what they're going to say, so they can listen to others as they talk.

• You start! Break the ice and set the tone.

Wear a Service Lens and Help Others Wear It

We'd like to introduce this tool with a true story that illustrates why wearing a service lens is so essential:

Recently one of the authors witnessed an upsetting hospital incident between a security guard and the mother of a baby about to go for surgery. Mom parked in a no-parking zone outside the front door of the hospital and across the driveway from a pharmacy. A hospital security guard approached her and said, "You can't park there!"

Mom explained, "I'm taking my baby for surgery and I've got to stop in the pharmacy for a minute."

The guard repeated, "You can't park here. You'll have to go to a lot."

Mom said, with panic in her voice, "I'm already late and I've got to get my baby to surgery."

The guard repeated, "Well, you can't park here!"

Leaving her baby in the backseat, Mom headed toward the pharmacy. The security guard walked over to her car and stuck a sticker on the side window. Mom saw this and yelled, "*What are you doing!*"

He responded, "Putting a no-parking sticker on your car because you can't park here."

Now irate, Mom yelled, "You get that sticker *off* my car. My baby's sick and I'll just be a minute."

In a harsh tone, the guard said, "I warned you that you can't park here and I'm not taking the sticker off!"

The conflict escalated. Mom proceeded to yell at the guard, call him names, and threaten his job. Through it all, the guard repeated, "I'm *not* taking that sticker off your car!" Enraged, Mom came at the guard as if to hit him, and the guard stalked across the street into another building. All this time, as Mom became more and more infuriated, the baby was shrieking in the car, and patients and families in the front lobby were all ears listening to the altercation.

Suddenly, coincidentally, an administrator arrived on the scene, got a quick lowdown about what had happened, and approached Mom, who was, at that moment, shrieking toward the building the guard entered, "I'll get you fired if it's the last thing I do!"

The administrator approached Mom, who immediately began shrieking at the administrator, too, insisting that she fire the guard immediately.

In a determined and calm fashion, the administrator said, "I really want to know what happened so I can help you. Will you please tell me what happened?" She had to say this more than once because Mom was so very upset and still ranting. Eventually, Mom sputtered out bits of the story.

While getting the gist, the administrator maintained eye contact with Mom and while she did, she began—without calling attention to it—to peel away at the sticker on the window. Worried that Mom was too upset to drive, the administrator kept the conversation going, apologizing for the sticker and for the guard's behavior, and asking if she could at this point do anything to help Mom and baby get what they needed and get to their surgery appointment.

Finally, Mom calmed down a bit. The two exchanged names and phone numbers and agreed to have a follow-up conversation.

Later, in a conversation between the author and the administrator, the administrator interpreted what had happened. She said, "The guard was following the rules. Preventing people from parking there—that's what he thought his job was at that moment. Meanwhile, Mom had a sick baby—which traumatizes any parent—and in the midst of her efforts to get her baby what she needed, the guard put that sticker on her car. Mom felt not only violated because of that sticky thing being put on her car (with a reprimand on it), but she also felt distraught that the guard had such disregard for her in this traumatic time with her baby. If only he had not put that sticker there, it wouldn't have happened. And once he did put it there, seeing her upset state, he should have removed the sticker as quickly as possible, apologizing all the while. That incident shows why we need to focus on service in a deliberate and visible way here. Our service is so good in so many ways. The fact is, this guard is a wonderful guy, as is his boss, the head of security. They care about service, but no doubt, they never had a conversation about what to do when policy and customer needs conflict. This guard thought that he needed to enforce policy in this case, even though doing so created such phenomenal distress for this mom and her sick baby. We need every manager to have conversations with his or her staff about the heart of the job and what to do when policies and patient needs conflict. In so many cases, staff should set policies aside unless doing so creates serious risks."

You need to have these kinds of conversations with staff, so that they can make decisions about how best to serve customers in tough situations—for instance, when policies suggest doing otherwise. These conversations are key since staff will fail customers unnecessarily because they don't see this as their primary job. We need to help staff make connections between service and their jobs when we are giving feedback, when orienting new employees, when doing performance reviews, and when discussing tasks and priorities—in every conversation.

This tool will help you look at your work world through a service lens so you can identify and take advantage of every opportunity to do the following:

- Remind staff about service.
- Highlight their importance to customer service and satisfaction.
- Coach them on service.
- Give feedback about their behavior and its effects on customers.
- In every other way, connect what they're doing to your service mission.

Method

The key to this tool is using every opportunity you can find to talk about and reinforce service and the critical role that impressing customers plays in shaping the future of your service and staff.

1. Make sure every staff member knows his or her role and potential contribution to the big picture of providing impressive service. Define roles in terms of service, and push staff to articulate their own service roles. Discuss with each and every staff member what his or her job is, and make customers primary in these discussions. Pinpoint the tough situations and talk through alternatives that work for customers without creating unacceptable risks for the organization. If people think that their job is anything but serving their customers, they undermine your efforts to create impressive customer service. For example, consider the job of the security guard in our story. Before focusing on service, he would have described his job very differently than after his organization focused on service.

Security Guard	
Old Job Description	New Job Description
I'm here to • Maintain a safe environment • Protect the assets of the organization • Enforce policies	I'm here to • Maintain a safe environment for patients and staff • Protect people from threats to their safety • Maintain a calm atmosphere that gives everyone who comes here a sense of security and a feeling that they're in good hands

2. When you react to specific behaviors that bother you about staff, talk to them about the implications for service and customer satisfaction. Describe the staff behavior that you see as problematic because of its effect on customers. Then, point out its impact on customers. For instance, try the following:

—Here's what I saw or heard about (describe the behavior).

—"I'm concerned about this because of its effects on your customers, namely _____.

—Here's an example:

Situation	Old Way	New Way
Employee arrives late habitually.	Supervisor says, "Your lateness is a problem!"	Supervisor says, "Your lateness creates delays for customers and places undue burdens on coworkers who need to stand in for you to serve your customers."
In an inpatient setting, employee fails to answer patients' call lights quickly.	Supervisor says, "You've got to respond faster. You take too long."	Supervisor says, "Patients become anxious, upset, and sometimes panicky when you take this long. This interferes with their healing and peace of mind, and their impression of us as responsive caregivers."

Employee spends too much time on personal calls.	Supervisor says, "You spend too much time on personal calls instead of working."	Supervisor says, "When you tie up the line with personal calls, customers are kept on hold because the line is busy. They get frustrated and annoyed with us and dissatisfied with our service."
Employee is slow to show up to answer patient call and says, "I'm sorry about the delay. We're really short-staffed since our recent layoffs. There aren't enough staff to do everything that needs doing."	Supervisor says nothing to employee because supervisor thinks, "Staff are right. We really *are* short-staffed!"	Supervisor confronts employee and says such comments are unacceptable because of their impact on customers. Patients lose confidence in the team and the organization. Supervisor needs to talk with staff about better, yet still honest, approaches, such as, "I'm so sorry you had to wait. I was helping another patient and it took a lot of time. Now I'm here and want to give you the help and time that you need."

3. When you react to specific behaviors that please you about staff, talk to them about the implications for service and customer satisfaction. The same point applies here. Connect positive contributions to effects on customers, too. For instance, "I really appreciated your fitting in that woman who came without the appointment. I appreciated it because it meant she wouldn't have to make another trip here. And I'm sure she appreciates you and us for that. That's one more satisfied customer you've created."

 Tips

- You need to strengthen your own service lens in order to do this. And you need to sharpen your skills at articulating the impact of behavior on customers. The good news is that the more you sharpen your lens and verbal skills, the easier it gets; and it will begin to come naturally without you having to remind yourself to do it.

- Especially when preparing to confront destructive behavior with a negative impact on customers, practice on friends and invite their feedback, so you can really explain what the problem is in terms of customer impact.

Focus on Service Improvement One Behavior at a Time

The tools in the previous section were designed to help you mainstream your service focus into everyday interactions, meetings, discussions, and decisions. That's your ultimate goal. It's too difficult to have to create programs and activities all the time to reinforce impressive service. The real challenge is to internalize your service focus into your bloodstream so that it affects your goals, interactions, relationships, decisions, and concerns all day, every day. Probably the best way to do this is by focusing attention and energy on one behavior at a time for a reasonable period of time (for example, one to four months depending on its complexity), so that this behavior becomes second nature to your staff.

Why focus on one behavior at a time? Good question. Here are some answers:

- It's easier to focus on one behavior than to focus on many; and it's not overwhelming. When you issue a long list of behaviors (which is inevitable if you are being thorough), staff may feel overwhelmed by the long list. No one is capable of absorbing and internalizing all of these behaviors at once. That's why it can be powerful to focus on one behavior at a time and help people develop the awareness, skills, and focus needed to effectively integrate that behavior as a habit in their everyday performance.
- It takes time to really improve a behavior and integrate it into your everyday actions and work. It takes time to go beyond surface improvements and internalize the change. There is more opportunity to learn and have the learning stick if we focus people's attention on one important behavioral goal, not many behaviors at once.

- Staff get better at changing behavior over time when they proceed one behavior at a time, and we provide a behavior change process for developing staff excellence. Once your team engages in this process, they start to learn the process and not just the behavior. As they move to the second behavioral goal and then the third, they find themselves getting better and better at the process. They proceed more easily, with the need for less planning. Over time, because the process becomes familiar, they find it easier to change the next behavior and the next.

Although these are compelling arguments, this approach does run the risk of trying your patience. Decide ahead of time that you will be patient. Sometimes, work teams develop a set of key service behaviors and the boss is so relieved to have these behaviors identified that he or she wants everyone to uphold every behavior right away. That's too much. It works so much better to focus everyone on one behavior at a time, in depth, and to install that behavior as habit before moving on to the next. Each behavior then gets the attention, skill building, and reinforcement required to make it crystal clear and routine.

Getting Started

Start by introducing the concept of improving one behavior at a time to your team, and engage them in selecting your first behavioral goal. But wait! Before you do, you need to believe in this approach so that you can effectively promote it. Ask yourself the following questions:

- Why do I really believe in this approach?
- How will it make a difference to staff and to customers?
- Why do I think that we will be able to be successful?
- What do I see as my role and my team's role in the process?

Think through these issues so you can make a convincing case for this approach. Also, think about the behaviors that you believe your team might well pursue first, and consider how open you are to their opinions and suggestions. If you already have a behavior in mind that you feel strongly about, admit this to your team. It isn't wise to go through the process with a behavior that you didn't believe needed attention. Also, it doesn't make sense to hide your feelings. Ideally, upon thinking this through, you'll realize that many behaviors would be appropriate as the first to pursue, and you'll invite your staff to select the first one they want to strengthen.

One Step at a Time: The Big Picture

Here's a tool you can use to introduce the one-behavior-at-a-time approach to your staff and to engage them in selecting your first behavioral goal. This approach will give staff an opportunity to learn about the steps in ironing out details and logistics, and it will guide their choices for the first behavior change initiatives.

Method

1. Introduce the one-behavior-at-a-time approach to your team by sharing your enthusiasm and commitment to the process. Post on a flipchart or pass out characteristics of the process, and use this visual aid to walk through your main arguments for the one-goal-at-a-time approach.

Improving Service Behaviors One Behavior at a Time

This process is	This process is not
• A long-term effort • A way for us to make improvements without getting overwhelmed • A way for everyone to get involved, rather than a few people or a team	• A Band-Aid or "program" • A way to punish the group because we are in trouble

2. Add items that address some of the concerns you know your staff have.
3. Provide your team with an overview of the steps in the process, so that they will see that this is not just a pep talk, but an introduction to serious work together to make improvements. Convey an open-minded, experimental attitude, emphasizing that

you want everyone to help develop and improve the process over time, since you know people will find kinks in it.

4. Ask the group to talk about what they like about what they've heard so far and to bring up any questions or concerns they have at this point. Capture these on a flipchart, answering any questions as they come up.

5. Now you're ready to choose the first behavioral goal. Ask the group to think of the criteria they could use to pick the first behavior. List these on a flipchart.
   —Is behavior important to customers?
   —Is it in need of improvement?
   —Does it involve everyone on the team?
   —Do staff and leaders care about it?
   —Does it bother us when we hear that we're relatively weak on this?
   —Is it something within our power to change?

6. Create a decision matrix with the criteria along the top and room for a list of alternative behaviors in the left-hand column. Then rate the importance each alternative behavior would have to various groups. The matrix would look something like this:

Possible Behaviors (1 = not very important, 2 = somewhat important, 3 = very important)					
	Important to customers?	Needs improvement?	Involves everyone on team?	Within our power to change?	Total
Greet warmly					
Respond quickly					
Maintain confidentiality					
Explain fully					
Be a telephone pro					

Ask the staff to identify behaviors they would like to work on and write them in the left-hand column of your grid.

7. Give everyone a copy of the grid to fill out, giving each behavior a low, medium, or high rating on each criterion you established as important. If you have a very large team, you might need to collect these forms, tally them, and reconvene the group to discuss the results. If you have a smaller group, do a quick tally and see which behavior wins right there at the meeting.

8. Wrap up the meeting with a discussion of the chosen behavior and ways people believe team members can improve on it.

9. Explain the next steps, specifically the planning process that will take place to map out the team's approach to improving the behavior significantly.

Tips

- The purpose of this upfront meeting is to excite your team about the one-behavior-at-a-time process and build their confidence that by using it, they can make a difference.
- Emphasize that they will be involved every step of the way.

Move on to Planning Your Approach

Beware! Don't fall into the trap of thinking you have to do the planning yourself. Consider these possibilities:

- If your staff is small, engage everyone in planning the approach.
- If your team is too large for that (and most are), form a subteam to develop every aspect of your approach to the selected behavior. For the next behavior selected, form a different subteam with at least one continuity person who served on the previous subteam. This enables an experienced planning subteam member to bring their experience forward to plan for the next behavior. Hold a planning meeting. This subteam's first job would be to plan the first staff meetings in which they introduce the behavioral goal and approach to their coworkers.
- Some people also elect service representatives for different work teams, and these reps meet as the planning team for all the behaviors selected for pursuit, one behavior at a time.

The One-Behavior-at-a-Time Improvement Process

This process has nine steps, many of which can be done quite quickly.

1. Raise awareness of this behavior among staff. Focus all eyes upon it.
2. For that behavior, examine the gap between current reality and impressive performance.
3. Set goals and targets.
4. Remove obstacles or minimize their impact.
5. Develop job-specific scripts and protocols as needed.
6. Enhance staff skills.
7. Get feedback on how well people are doing and inform the staff.
8. Recognize positive performance.
9. Institute ongoing monitoring and feedback to maintain the gains and trigger further improvement.

Each step is explained in detail in the sections that follow. Once your team gets familiar with what's involved at each step, they will be able to move much more quickly and efficiently through the steps when they pursue future behavioral goals. They'll get better and speedier at the process.

Step 1: Raise Awareness

In step 1, you will raise awareness of the behavior among staff. The challenge here is to get everyone focused on the same objective. You need staff to understand the following:

- Why this behavior is so important to our customers
- Why we chose this behavior
- The opportunities we have to improve
- What's in this for all of us if we do improve

If you skip this step and jump immediately into improvement activities, you jeopardize the process and the likelihood that you'll get results. Members of your team view service behaviors very differently. Working together with you, they need to establish and share a common vision as well as a common frame of reference related to the behavior at hand. Everyone needs to be reminded that the pursuit is for all, not just some. Everyone needs to see that they have room to improve and that if everyone participates, it will add up to a noticeable improvement in behavior and have a significant effect on customer satisfaction. Also, you and fellow believers in customer service need another chance to challenge the skeptics who say it won't work and it can't be done.

Tell your team that you're now going to initiate a variety of activities designed to help them become clearer about what it takes to become impressive at the chosen behavior and to develop a clear rationale for doing so.

 ## Scavenger Hunt

This tool has three purposes:

1. To raise team awareness of the importance of the chosen behavior for customers and for each other
2. To help staff see the difference between good and great with regard to the behavior in a variety of settings
3. To develop a common language related to the behavior

Method

1. Give staff one or two weeks to observe other people demonstrating the behavior. They are to look for people who epitomize excellence in this behavior and also those who miss opportunities. These people can be from within your service, department, or organization, or from outside of the organization in local businesses or other industries. Invite staff to work alone or with a partner on this. Ask them to use the following chart to help them record their observations.

Observe! Find Examples of the Behavior in Other People

Situation:

What staff did or said:

What staff did not do or did not say:

How this made me feel:

What I liked:

What I think could have been improved:

2. At the next staff meeting, invite people to share their experiences and look for the common themes and examples.
3. Ask the group to make a statement about what they learned from the experience.

Tips

- Make sure that your team talks about the different ways they can observe the behaviors.
- Encourage them to discuss where they can go to find people doing this behavior, as well as what they might have to do to elicit (or provoke) the behavior from people. For example, if your team is working on the behavior to be flexible, give people ideas about how they might present staff with an opportunity to be flexible and/or provide people with choices. They could go to a restaurant and request food that's not on the menu. They could present a

challenge to the same individual, by having a dietary restriction, to see what the person would say and do. Brainstorm possibilities with staff before you send them on their hunt.

- Consider assigning people a number of examples they need to find. And encourage them to look for positive as well as negative examples.
- When you process the information, make sure that you do the following:

  —Push people to be very specific. The learning is in the details. This is important for staff to begin to understand. The entire process of moving from good to impressive is about paying attention to the details.

  —Ask, "How did the person you observed make you feel as a customer by what they did and said?" Push this discussion so that your staff see the effects and consequences of demonstrating or failing to demonstrate the behavior.

 ### We Are the Best

Here's another tool for awareness raising that helps staff grapple with what it takes to be impressive and recognize what it takes to be seen as leaders in demonstrating the chosen behavior.

Method

1. Divide the group into smaller groups (about four to six people), and ask small groups to respond to this question: "We have just won the service award in our industry for being the best at [chosen behavior]. Think about what we had to do and say to our customers and each other that put us in the limelight."
2. Ask each group to think about specific things that staff had to do and say to win this very prestigious award.
3. Have groups share their ideas with the whole group. See which group generates the most examples and suggestions.
4. Then ask the group to think about what it would take to make their fantasies a reality. Ask, "What would have to happen for our team to win the award?" (They might mention such things as a commitment from everyone, direction from leadership, a

common vision, and a way to hold themselves and the team accountable.)

Tip

- Push your team to picture the impressive level of behavior. If they can't stretch their concept of excellence, many will have trouble acknowledging that they have room for improvement. The result is they'll feel exempt while they expect others to improve.

Ongoing Visual Reminders

The activities described above are all interactive ways to help your team understand why the chosen behavior is important and what they need to consider to improve on this behavior for their customers' sake. Use also visual and written methods of keeping your team's focus on the chosen behavior. Many methods accomplish this, some of which create great opportunities for staff creativity.

Method

1. *Poster of the month:* Ask staff to contribute ideas for posters and be responsible for hanging a different poster each month to reinforce the behavior in focus. Consider having a poster contest as one way to generate great posters.
2. *Customer service behavior banner:* Invite someone with some graphic design skills to create a banner and hang it in a very public area.
3. *Cartoons and jokes:* Ask staff to bring in cartoons that illustrate the importance of the service behavior. Display these on a bulletin board or hang them in a public area. If you don't have a bulletin board, create a space on the wall and decorate it in some way so that you are not just tacking a piece of paper on a blank wall.
4. *Job aids:* Make small written reminders of any protocols you develop related to the behavior. Also, put these on tent cards in your lounge/lunch area or on bulletin boards.
5. *Signs or fliers:* Hang nicely formatted signs or fliers in public areas so that your external customers know you are focusing on

a particular behavior. It impresses customers when they learn that your team is working on raising service standards. After all, it is for their sake! Have your team develop ways to inform customers about your behavioral goal. Here's an example:

Example of a Reminder Visible to Staff and Customers

Dear Customers:

We are working on enhancing our customer service for your sake. We have identified customer service behaviors important to our customers and are highlighting one each month/quarter. We would like your help in letting us know how we're doing.

This month's customer service behavior is _____.

Please let us know how we're doing. Your satisfaction is our priority.

Tips

- Don't feel compelled to create visual reminders yourself. Involve your team. Perhaps form an awareness subcommittee that invites and considers suggestions and takes responsibility for implementing them throughout your campaign.
- You'll find some staff who love doing this kind of work and are very talented. Open it up to your people and see who meets the challenge. Position it boldly as important to the team. Show staff that you not only welcome but value their participation and contributions.

Step 2: Examine the Gap

Now that staff are attuned to the importance of the behavior, help them identify the gap between an impressive level of performance on that behavior and their current level of performance.

What Would They Say?

This tool will help the team evaluate how they feel they're doing on the behavior, specifically identifying the gap between current performance and the impressive level of performance.

Method

1. Give each member the following worksheet:

What do you wish customers would say about how well this team exhibits this behavior?	What do you think customers would really say?

2. Ask staff to form pairs and do this: Imagine that you are over-hearing two customers talking about our service and how we are doing related to the behavior we've chosen to improve. What, in the ideal, do you hope or wish they were saying? Ask people to focus at first on the ideal, not current reality.

3. Give the pairs several minutes to discuss and take notes on their discussions.

4. Ask the partners to share their ideas with the larger group, looking for common themes and opinions. Push the group to come up with some very specific quotes and examples of what people could be saying about this team's demonstration of the behavior at hand.

5. Ask the pairs to join with another pair, making up groups of four. Ask these groups to think about current reality and to address the question, "What are customers really saying about us as it relates to the behavior we're working on?" Again, ask the groups to discuss, take notes, and finally share their results with the larger group.

6. Record the findings on a flipchart.

7. Compare the two lists (what our customers are really saying versus what we wish they were saying). Ask people to identify the gaps between the ideal and the reality.

8. Summarize: It seems that we're doing some things very well and yet we do have some room for improvement. That's why we've chosen this behavior as our goal. Our goal is to have our

customers talking about us in real life the way we wished they did when we talked about our ideal.

9. Finally, ask your team to look over the lists and choose one aspect of the behavior on which they think they can make a difference (a simple aspect is fine) and ask them to commit to working on this as a team.

Tips

- Push staff to identify missed opportunities because these opportunities reflect the gaps between current reality and optimal performance.
- This tool provides a backdrop for rational goal setting. Don't skip it!

Step 3: Set Goals and Targets

Now that staff have identified the gap between current reality and an impressive level of performance, ask people to set goals for the team.

Where Should We Aim?

With this tool, you can pinpoint specific improvement goals for the team that advance people to the impressive level of behavior.

Method

1. Ask staff to revisit the gap between current reality and an impressive level of performance and to identify the following:
   —The subgoals that will lead them to their overall goal of reaching an impressive level of performance
   —The precise standard they want to reach

2. Start by brainstorming possible subgoals or routes to the overall goal of achieving an impressive level of behavior. For instance, if the overall behavior you're focusing on is "Keep the noise down" (because a quiet, calm environment is therapeutic), subgoals might include the following:
   —Move close to coworkers when talking, so you don't have to yell.

—Take initiative to oil squeaky door hinges and equipment wheels.

—Use overhead paging system for emergencies only.

3. Now, turn these subgoals into targets by setting a standard for each that will require a stretch or change in people's behavior. For example, for the "Keep it quiet" behavioral goal, standards might be the following:

—Replace *all* (100 percent) of the yelling down the hall with close face-to-face conversations.

—Oil (and reduce the squeaks on) 10 wheel or door hinges a day and institute a preventive maintenance schedule that prevents all squeaks by [a certain date].

—Reduce the number of overhead pages per day from 120 to 15 or fewer.

4. Ask the team to help you complete this worksheet to pull together their statement of goals and targets:

Our overall goal is to _____.

To bring this behavior to an impressive level, everyone individually needs to _____

_____.

And our team as a whole needs to _____.

Breaking this down into its component parts, our specific targets are the following:

_____

_____

_____

Tips:

• Push people to pin down the standard you want to reach as a team. Make this standard quantitative, which takes some ingenuity. The routes to achieving your overall behavioral goal need to be very clear and observable, not conceptual or attitudinal.

• Encourage identification of goals for the team and goals for the individuals on the team. The fact is, if an individual drags down the standard, the impression customers have of the team falters.

Step 4: Remove Obstacles or Minimize Their Impact

So far, we've talked about why it makes sense to focus on improving a key service behavior. It is hoped that by now you see how to enlist your staff's energies and use their input as well as customer input to set some ambitious behavioral standards and targets. Now consider the obstacles or what's in the way of reaching your targets.

Why focus on barriers? Here are a few reasons:

• You don't want to set your team up for failure.
• You don't want barriers or brick walls to frustrate your team so that they ultimately quit trying to achieve the improvement at hand. There are ways to help your team identify barriers to their behavioral goals and take responsibility for fixing them. The twist? These initiatives relate to *one* aspect of service, to *one* very specific behavior.

You'll find several approaches in this book in chapter 4, "Remove Barriers so Staff Can Serve Customers," which you can adapt for your behavior-of-the-month/quarter campaigns. And here are other ideas specific to this end.

 ### What's in the Way?

This tool has three purposes:

1. To develop a common understanding of the barriers staff see as preventing them from improving on or making it difficult for them to improve on the targeted behavior
2. To generate ideas about how to remove or reduce these barriers or obstacles
3. To help staff take responsibility for eliminating the more obvious and frustrating obstacles

Method

1. Begin by discussing barriers and obstacles in the broad sense. Let staff know that not only are you committed to eliminating obstacles, but that as a group they have demonstrated the power to reduce obstacles to goals they've set in the past. Ask people, "What are barriers or obstacles that you've seen us eliminate or reduce to make our services better in the past? How have these efforts made a difference to you and to our customers?" Build people's confidence in their track records of reducing obstacles.

2. Now focus your team on the chosen behavior of the month/quarter, and the related standards and the targets. Tell people that the purpose of this meeting is to get clear about the obstacles that impede their ability to reach the target (their improvement goals).

   —Ask the group to brainstorm very specific everyday things that present a challenge to or pose obstacles to demonstrating an impressive level of the behavior at hand. As people brainstorm, write their responses on Post-Its, one issue per stickie.

   —When the group has run out of ideas, ask several people to put the stickies on the wall and ask the group to build an affinity (cluster) diagram. That is, without talking, have them move the stickies around until they form categories or clusters of related ideas. They might identify categories such as policy issues, equipment issues, people issues, team relationship issues, communication issues, systems issues, and so on.

   —When your team finally has the stickies in the right categories, give each small group one category to work with. For their category, ask the small groups to sort the issues into the following groups:

   –Quick fixes: Actions we can accomplish right away

   –Breakthrough barriers: Accomplishments that would make a big difference if we could only figure out how to achieve them

   –Unpreventable barriers: Those we might not be able to fix, but we can develop ways to work around them or minimize their effects.

3. Once the small groups have prioritized their issues, ask them to present their findings to the whole team.

4. The whole team looks over the quick fixes to see which ones they want to act on right away or down the line. Acknowledge that even though many might be quick-fix items, people have finite energy to spend. A quick way to prioritize is to have the teams rate the issues on a 1- to 4-point scale for each of a small number of criteria.

   —How serious a problem is it to customers and to staff?
   —How easy is it to solve?

5. Pick the high-scoring items that may be easier to solve or address.

6. Have your team use a similar process for the remaining categories. This enables people to focus on high-priority breakthroughs, as well as the unpreventables.

7. You are now ready to ask your team to commit to obstacles they will tackle. Look at the issues with a high score. A good way to move into the next phase is to have individuals think about the kinds of projects that they personally would like to work on. Ask everyone to think about being either a resource or a full member of some improvement work team. Remember, because many of these ideas will be quite simple, you're not asking for gigantic investments of time or full-scale continuous quality improvement (CQI) teams.

8. If there's time, divide into work groups (if not, do this at your next meeting). Have groups meet briefly to discuss the improvement goals they've set. Give each small team 15 minutes to respond to these questions:

   —Why do we feel this obstacle or barrier needs to be removed?
   —What will it take for us to do so?
   —What support, resources, or information will we need to help us?
   —What can the entire team expect from us and by when?

9. The small groups then share their plans with the larger group and invite feedback or input from coworkers.

10. Set a date for the next meeting.

11. Groups get to work.

Tips

- The success of this approach depends on your group's openness to owning and solving problems together. Many groups don't think that it's their job. They want their boss to be the fixer! That's a problematic attitude. If your team shares this attitude, you will need to do more groundwork related to what their jobs entail as service providers. This job needs to include getting involved in solving service problems and with that, reducing obstacles to impressive service.

- Success depends also on your team's track record at solving problems and overcoming obstacles. You can't do anything about the past except learn from it, but you may have to go back and revisit with them some of their past experiences to see what helped and hurt in past problem-solving efforts, so you can together identify what needs to be different this time.

- Finally, your team's success depends on their finding time to work on these improvement projects. Many will wonder, "I'm so busy. How can I possibly take on one other thing?" You'll need to figure out with people how they can spring loose to work on these improvement projects, or indeed they won't. You might need to rearrange schedules or pay overtime or arrange coverage for each other so people will have time to work together. What won't work is for you to say, "You and your groups will need to work that out on your own."

Step 5: Develop Job-Specific Scripts and Protocols

So, now you've raised awareness, identified goals and targets, and identified and started to tackle obstacles to reaching an impressive level of performance related to your behavior of the month/quarter. The next step is to get very clear about how to translate *impressive* into scripts and protocols that, when followed, ensure consistency at this impressive level.

Let's say your behavioral goal for the month/quarter is to greet customers in ways that reflect warmth, hospitality, and helpfulness. Behavioral subgoals or targets related to this might be to make eye contact, smile, introduce yourself to customers, and offer to help them 100 percent of the time.

To help staff move to an impressive level of customer service, involve them in developing for each specific job greeting protocols or scripts that contain all of the elements of a greeting that their customers find impressive. Here's a simple script for a front desk receptionist: "Hello! Welcome to Jones Associates! I'm Helen Harris. May I have your name please?"

Protocol and Script Work Session

This tool has two goals:

1. To identify for each job in your service any scripts and protocols needed to pinpoint the words and deeds key to an impressive level of behavior
2. To equip staff with job aids to remind them of the scripts and protocols.

Method

1. Form small groups by position. If you have only one person in certain positions, have them team up together.
2. Ask the small groups to serve as consultants to one another, focusing on one position at a time. The task is to identify those targeted behaviors that involve several actions or words. These are behaviors that can be well supported by a script or protocol.
3. Imagine that you are programming a robot to demonstrate an impressive level of performance on the behaviors at hand. Program the robot. Develop in writing a protocol and/or script that details exactly what the robot should do and exactly what the robot should say to behave in an impressive way.
4. Have the small groups then swap scripts and protocols with other groups to get feedback and invite suggested refinements.
5. The last step is to streamline the results and record them onto job aids (cards, guide sheets, or checklists) to be given to people in the specific job to remind them of the details that reflect impressive performance of the behavior at hand.

Tips

- Some staff will be better at script and protocol development than others. Consider the alternative of having small groups brainstorm elements of scripts and protocols for each job and then have a small design team polish these into well-articulated, visually appealing job aids.

- Refer to chapter 2 for more details on how to develop scripts and protocols.

Step 6: Enhance Staff Skills

Now people know which behaviors they're supposed to exhibit in very specific terms. But can they exhibit them? Do they have the skill? You can safely expect that staff skills related to the standard of the month/quarter will vary. Some people will want to uphold the standard, but their past habits are not up to speed. It's critical to take the time to help them build their skills, so that they can be successful.

You've probably noticed that there's no chapter in this book about training. This is not an oversight. Many customer service initiatives have focused primarily on training and, quite frankly, are unsuccessful because of this. Why? The training was done out of context. It didn't relate directly enough to people's real work. Also, frequently the training was disconnected from performance expectations and accountability. People might learn to perform a skill better in the training environment, but then, they could return to their work site and act the same way as always with no consequence.

Although we built training components into every chapter linked to the strategy presented, training is critical in this section. If there's one place you and staff can greatly benefit from training, it's in the service of pursing excellence, one behavior at a time.

- You've chosen a specific behavioral focus, so the training can be very targeted and skill specific.
- You have clarified that this is for everyone, that everyone is expected to engage in the behavior at an impressive level, and that this training is a support for people along the way.
- You're set up for success because you're building feedback methods for monitoring performance and giving the results to your team. All the conditions are right to make training important and effective.

The approach we're recommending here is what we call 20-minute skill builders. These are short exercises within the context of each staff meeting or in-service session in which you help people sharpen their skills.

Use your existing steering committee or form one to develop the agenda of skill builders and to line up the facilitators or other resource people you need to run them. Here are a few ideas to get you started:

- Each idea should be simple to facilitate and shouldn't require fancy equipment.
- Each idea should work with any group size.
- Each idea should adapt to groups with every level of skill.

 ### Fine-Tuning Service Behaviors

Here's a good basic approach to skill building that will help staff see that getting better is about paying attention to the details of impressive performance related to the behavior of the quarter/month.

Method

1. At a staff meeting, ask your team to think about common situations in which they have opportunities to demonstrate the behavior at hand. Narrow this list down to a few opportunities that most of the group share.
2. Ask people to describe their typical behavior in these situations.
3. Help people define what it takes to move from the typical way they demonstrate these behaviors to the exceptional way that would wow their customers.
4. In small groups, ask the staff to look over the examples and identify one or two things that everyone could do to move from good to impressive. Have the groups share their results with the whole group and ask for group commitment to engage in these new behaviors in the coming weeks when the typical opportunities arise.

 Tips

- Don't get too, too ambitious. Work in a very specific way on one or two things that all staff can do to improve behavior.
- View this as a chance to tend to the small details that make a

difference as well as a way to ensure consistency in the team's approach to typical situations.

Isn't There a Better Way?

This tool can help staff identify red flag statements that turn off customers or provoke defensiveness.

Method

1. Introduce the concept of red flag statements. Red flag statements are words and phrases that staff might say that send out a clear message to customers that staff don't care about them or their needs. Often these words and phrases are short, unconscious throwaway lines. But they can have a walloping negative impact on customers.

2. Ask people to turn to a partner and share a time when they were on the receiving end of a red flag statement—at work or elsewhere. Share a few of these then in the large group.

3. Now, focusing on the behavior of the month/quarter, ask staff to think about typical situations and possible red flag statements that could get them offtrack. And finally, ask people to state the positive alternative for that same situation. For example, let's say the behavior of the month is "Be flexible." Use a chart like this to get your team's thoughts on paper:

Situation	Red Flag Statement	Positive Alternative
I need an appointment with a specialist.	We don't do that here.	I'm not familiar with this kind of specialist. So let me call our referral service and see if they can help you.
I want to bring my children to visit.	Our policy doesn't permit that.	While children are not permitted on this floor because of safety concerns, let me see if I can locate a room where they might visit with you.

4. See if your team will agree to help each other avoid these statements by adopting a subtle signal that they will all use if they hear a coworker use a red flag statement, such as the word *gong* said quietly.

Tips

- This is a simple, powerful activity that can take just a few minutes. It's an important one because it helps to stamp out negative behavior that people aren't aware is interfering with the behavior at hand.
- Come prepared to cite a few examples. If possible, own them. Say, "I have at times caught myself saying _____." This will make it safer for people to admit the red flag statements they use and hear.

Other 20-Minute Skill Builders

- Show the contrast between poor and impressive behavior: Put on skits (with props, costumes, and the like) of everyday situations in which people are living the chosen behavior to the hilt. Contrast this with skits in which people are violating the behavior outrageously.
- Discuss how the behavior relates to interactions with a specific customer group: Have a flipchart ready with that month's behaviors. Give staff members a customer category, that is, external (patient/family) or internal (physician/colleague) and ask them to identify the specific opportunities to uphold that behavior with that customer group. Then, divide people into pairs and, naming one opportunity at a time, have the pairs take turns practicing the behavior for their partner and inviting feedback.
- Demonstrate and clarify each of the subgoals related to the behavior of the month or quarter: Break staff up into the same number of miniteams as there are subgoals. Give each miniteam one subgoal and ask them to prepare a role play or skit (in 5 minutes) that shows how to demonstrate an impressive level of behavior related to it. Have each group perform their role play. After each, the facilitator invites comments about the behavior (what makes it hard, what makes it easy, what would help make it more effective) and then moves on to the next group for their role play.

- Share relevant information: Depending on the behavioral goal, there might be information that needs to shared. Bring in outside resources to help. For instance, when you address phone tactics, you might want to bring in your service areas telephone directory or resource people to provide a discussion on how to handle calls better. Or you might show and discuss a good videotape on the subject.
- Give staff an experience that will help them become more effective at the behavior. For instance, if you address a standard related to giving directions, have people bring in maps, or give tours during the meeting so staff learn how to give better directions.

Tips on Skill Builders

- The most important thing to remember about 20-minute skill-building sessions is that staff need improved skills and also reinforcement to extend impressive service to their customers day in and day out. Make sure that the skill-building sessions are continual. For instance, create a schedule for six months at a time, so that staff see the importance you place on reinforcing and improving their customer service performance.
- As each month moves along, make sure that sessions get better over time by having staff evaluate each session and suggest improvements. For instance, place a + and − at the top of a flipchart. Take two minutes to ask staff what worked about the meeting and what needs improvement so that the next team can take the ideas and build on them to make the next session even better.
- If you have staff serving as facilitators, make sure they get a great round of applause at the end of each session. Also meet with them to thank them and tell them specifically what they did that you think made a difference to this initiative.

Step 7: Get Feedback

Key to focusing all eyes on the behavior of the month/quarter is providing staff with feedback from their customers' perspectives. How well are staff performing this behavior? How effective are they? What is the impact on customers? By providing feedback with a rapid turnaround time, staff can make incremental improvements that build on each other to add up to significant behavior change.

 ## Survey on the Behavior of the Month/Quarter

This tool will help you solicit customer feedback about staff performance of the behavior of the month/quarter and provide this information quickly—in time to encourage staff to make further improvements.

Method

1. Develop a short customer survey related to the standard of the month—a short report card that gives staff feedback about their behaviors related to the standard of the month from their customers' perspectives.

Dear Customer,

This month we're focusing on improving the way we greet our customers and make them feel at home here. Please give us feedback about three quick questions related to how you were greeted today. This will help us improve our service.

1. Did staff greet you immediately when you arrived?
   Yes   No

2. Did the person who greeted you smile and say something welcoming?
   Yes   No

3. Did everyone who greeted you introduce themselves to you?
   Yes   No

Please give us any suggestions on how our staff can greet people more effectively:

Please place your completed form in the box on the front desk. Thank you very much!

And thanks for listening!

---

2. Have staff tally the results at the end of each week and circulate the group scores to people on the following Monday. Post the results for all to see and/or hold a staff meeting in which you ask the following:
   —What do you think about these results?
   —What can we do to raise our scores even higher?

Tips

- Rotate tallying responsibility, so no one staff member is doing all the tallying for more than a week.
- Keep the surveys short and to the point. Focus one question on each subgoal of the behavior at hand.
- Leave room for comments.

Variations

- Provide staff with notepads headed with "A bit of feedback about (the behavior)" with a format for constructive feedback. Urge people to write these notes to each other in the spirit of helping each other make the team's service quality impressive. Here's a sample format:

Dear (coworker's name),

I noticed you (name the behavior).

The results were (name the consequences, effects).

A suggestion I have is (make a suggestion).

- Place a dinner bell or soothing gong in a central area. Encourage staff to ring it when they see behavior needing improvement. The sound should trigger everyone to ask themselves, "What did I just do? Am I living up to our standards?" It can be rung once if improvement is needed and can be rung twice if the person/people have given great service.

- If staff are good-natured and open, use a squeeze toy (such as a rubber duck). Have someone start with it and give it to a colleague if they need improvement on that month's standard/behavior. That person then keeps the rubber duck until they see someone else who needs improvement, and then they pass it on to them. Hopefully, this will make people be more alert to what they are doing and catch themselves violating the standard.

Tips

- Direct feedback can be powerful and very helpful to this process. Talk about and have the team practice how to give each other feedback using the standards and behaviors. Have someone show how to give feedback to enhance the relationship and teamwork and how not to give feedback.
- Keep your feedback methods light, while at the same time making the point that feedback is key to raising the bar on the behavior of the month/quarter.

Step 8: Recognize Positive Performance

Hopefully by now, you've seen significant improvement because people are not only keenly aware of the behavior of the month/quarter, but they've also had job aids, skill practice, and feedback to help them reach an impressive level of performance.

Behavior of the Month/Quarter Recognition

This tool will help you appreciate and reinforce people for their progress toward impressive performance, as well as build into your standard process methods of recognizing and celebrating their progress.

Method

1. Starting the first day of the month, give each staff member two coupons to a local ice-cream parlor. When they see a coworker display the behavior in an impressive way, they give that person a coupon. At the end of the month, the person with the most coupons receives special recognition during a staff meeting.

Have staff create an appreciation card that all customers can use to recognize staff for giving great service related to the standard of the month.

Dear Customer,

This month, this service team is focusing on consistently living this standard in our relationships with our customers.

Standard:

Related behaviors:

Please compliment a staff member you see living up to this standard by completing this note and dropping it in the box on the front desk. Thank you very much.

From (your name please) _____

Today, I saw a staff member named _____ behave in accord with your service standard of the month. Specifically, what they did was _____.

I appreciated this because _____.

Tips

- Engage your team in developing creative approaches to recognition. Staff can generate many other ideas, and they'll have fun doing this.
- Be a positive role model. Write appreciation notes to staff members who exemplify the behavior of the month/quarter.

Step 9: Institute Ongoing Monitoring and Feedback

By now, you will have seen big improvements. Unfortunately, staff run the risk of backsliding if they don't get feedback. This last step is key to maintaining your hard-won gains. Build into your ongoing "customer satisfaction monitoring methods" questions or items related to the behaviors you targeted for improvement, so you can give staff regular feedback about how they're doing. Also, build into your staff performance review process the behaviors staff worked so hard to improve.

The behavior of the month/quarter approach is your best hedge against overwhelming staff with too many expectations at a time. This approach also helps you to help staff focus and try for a higher level of performance, one behavior at a time, a doable process even in an atmosphere of stress and multiple demands.

Stop Speeding On to the Next Problem before You Appreciate Progress Already Made

So far we've described two ways to maintain your service focus. First, by mainstreaming your service focus or integrating it into everyday situations. And second, by focusing on service improvement one behavior at a time. A third overall approach to maintaining your service focus involves recognizing staff for their hard work and results when customers are happier and service is improving. This isn't easy because it requires you to stop speeding from one problem to another before you appreciate progress on the problem you just relieved.

Here are symptoms that indicate a need for you to focus in this area:

- Staff gripe about feeling unappreciated.
- People say, "We only hear about it when it's bad!"
- Staff groan about being overworked.
- Staff really extend themselves to serve their customers well.
- You feel frustrated that you can't pay staff more, because you think they deserve it.

If you nodded to many of these, you're not alone. Most managers yearn for better ways to recognize staff for their everyday contributions to great service.

Especially in today's stressful environment, it takes a lot of personal energy to serve customers well. It requires a person to bring their whole selves to work—not just their skills, but also their spirits and heart. People who do this (and many don't) not only deserve notice, but also genuine regard.

Most health care workers entered health care because they care. They wanted to have a job that allows them to help others. But then, in so many health care jobs, they find numerous barriers to providing good care and service: bureaucracy, work overload, equipment shortages, and much more. And the stresses inherent in today's health care environment distract people from their original missions. By recognizing people for the behavior they most value, you remind them of their service mission and they feel enhanced and less depleted by the stress inherent in their work.

Many managers, customers, and coworkers only give employees feedback when some aspect of their service disturbs them. People seem much more prone to give negative feedback than positive feedback. Employees feel like they are giving, giving, giving, and all they hear is what they do wrong—how they disappoint. By creating an atmosphere in which staff receive positive feedback and appreciation, you help them keep perspective. This feeds their sense of self-worth and sparks their energy to give even more of themselves.

Not the Same Old Thing

The old way is for the manager or supervisor to shoulder all the responsibility for giving recognition and appreciation. This is probably an artifact of the paternalistic way of managing, in which the manager sets the expectations, plans and controls the situation, gives the negative feedback and positive feedback, and essentially takes full responsibility for everyone's behavior. This is a heavy burden and, in today's environment, violates many employees' desires for latitude to act, empowerment, and shared responsibility for service design, problem solving, and outcomes.

What does this mean about recognition? It means that you as manager need to be only one of the sources of recognition, not the sole source.

- *Managers:* You are one important source of recognition and appreciation, and you might need to step up your own activity in that direction. But you are only one source.
- *The team:* When you establish the team as the driver of service quality, you need to create structures and opportunities to help the team be the dispenser of recognition for its own members. Coworkers and peers need to be the dispensers of recognition and appreciation for each other.
- *The individual:* Because people are so busy doing their own jobs, much customer service is never seen by peers or the boss. If the employee depends on recognition from peers and the boss, but their excellence is not observed, how can peers and the boss know to give recognition? What's the answer? You need to foster employee independence and create structures and opportunities that help employees recognize and appreciate their own acts of goodness toward customers. They will be perpetually starved for recognition if dependent on others to give it.
- *Customers:* And finally, you have a great opportunity to escalate recognition and appreciation of staff by creating ways to help customers give this to staff directly.

Here are four kinds of recognition tools that reinforce contributions to impressive service:

1. Tools that you as manager can use to recognize staff
2. Tools coworkers can use to recognize each other
3. Tools you can use to help staff appreciate their own service contributions
4. Tools you can provide to entice customers to give positive feedback directly to members of your team

Tools That You as Manager Can Use to Recognize Staff

You are in a powerful role as supervisor. Your perceptions of people's performance matter to your team. You influence them. By focusing recognition on your staff for their contributions to impressive service specifically, you can help to boost the quality of service and build staff gratification and morale all the while.

Try a mix of methods, not just one. Focus your power on recognizing people for their service behavior.

Verbal Recognition

Some people struggle to find the words to say thanks effectively. Here's a wonderful model that helps you find the words easily. This kind of staff recognition connects their service behavior with consequences for customers and also helps staff feel appreciated for their contributions.

Method

Deliver verbal thanks, whether in writing or aloud by following this model. The model calls for four steps to a great "Thanks!"

1. *Behavior:* Specifically, describe the service behavior you appreciated. For example, "I noticed or I heard that you _____."
2. *Impact:* Describe the impact—the consequences for the customer, the service's image, the organization, the mission. For example, "This had the effect of _____."
3. *Pinch of empathy:* Show an understanding that the employee had to undergo effort, or difficulties, or go out of their way to do what they did. For example, "I realize it's not easy to _____."
4. *Thanks:* Explicitly express your appreciation. For example, "Thank you. I really appreciate it, and I know your customers do, too."

Here are examples of the four-step model in action:

> By the way, Saundra, thank you for helping me to photocopy and collate the research proposal *(behavior)*. I doubt that I could have finished it on time without your help; you helped relieve the pressure I was feeling *(consequences/impact)*. I realize you had to set aside what you were working on to help me and that this might have increased the pressures on you *(pinch of empathy)*. I really do appreciate you for pitching in. You're a model of respect for internal customers *(thanks)!*

> Ann, I heard you made Sally Brown's high-risk delivery of her daughter a very positive experience for this frightened new mom. You paid undivided attention, showed warmth, caring, and strong support during a very traumatic time. I realize it

consumed lots of your time and energy. I really appreciate all
you did to make our service a symbol of hospitality!

Tips

- Have your team's service-behaviors list on hand as an aid. Connect their behavior to behaviors on this list to reinforce these
  behaviors and keep awareness high.
- Create a job aid for yourself that spells out the four-step
  model. Use it to be sure you include every key facet of effective feedback and recognition in your verbal messages. After a
  while, the four steps will become second nature (because
  you'll see how effective they are), and you will no longer need
  the job aid!
- Use the same model for writing thank-you notes to staff.

Congratulatory Banners

Visual recognition in the form of banners or posters is a good way
to post progress and good news for all to see.

Method
Hang visible congratulatory signs or banners in public places for
individuals or the team when they do something outstanding that
relates to your customer service commitment, such as the following:
reflecting behaviors well; getting accolades from customers; doing a
great job on a customer service project; reaching or exceeding a service target; or being creative and resourceful together in a crisis situation with customers.

Walk the Talk

You can demonstrate in your own behavior a customer service orientation toward your own staff.

Method
Some people might say this method goes without saying. We don't
think so, because so many managers don't do it naturally.

1. Greet your employees when you pass their desks or pass them in the hall. Call them by name and be willing to stop and talk. Express interest in their health, family, interests, and work.
2. When they are swamped, pitch in. Show that you value internal customer service, with you in the provider role and members of your team and colleagues in the customer role.
3. Look over your staff's service-behaviors list and identify opportunities when you can demonstrate these behaviors in your everyday interactions with staff. Do it.

Tips

- This is where your feet hit the pavement. To put it bluntly, go beyond lip service or rhetoric and practice what you preach!
- If you don't walk the service walk, you can expect resistance and cynicism among members of your team. People think, "If he or she doesn't, then why should I?"

Service Recognition Warm-Ups

Warm-ups like the ones described here can start staff meetings in ways that help staff recognize the positive service contributions of themselves and their peers.

Method

Do one of the following warm-ups per meeting:

1. Ask, "Since we last met, what good example of great service have you seen someone here provide?"
2. Thank someone there publicly for helping *you* out in a tough situation.
3. Brag about one example of great service that you provided since you saw each other last.
4. Commend the group on a service strength you noticed in the last week.

Tips

- Invite your staff to suggest other warm-ups.
- When you run out, start again, because the answers will differ.

- Be sure to participate yourself, too. Be a role model of willing participation and share your perceptions as well.

Tools Coworkers Can Use to Recognize Each Other

There's a great message in this approach. When you help staff recognize each other, you're creating a more egalitarian atmosphere. You're saying, "We are a team of people who appreciate each other" instead of, "I'm the boss and it's my recognition that counts."

Who's Good at What?

Involve your team in recognizing each other with this easy tool.

Method

1. Give each employee a list of all the employees on your team. Ask them to write one sentence next to each person's name about a positive example of service being offered by this person during the last week/month—an example with either internal or external customers that they appreciated. Ask people to be specific, since specific feedback—including positive feedback— is most meaningful to people.
2. Have people turn in all of their sheets to you. Compile all the comments about each person and return to each person the sheet that relates to them. You can make it easier by having staff type their entries into a computer.
3. The result: There will be a glow among your team members surrounding this activity, as people receive appreciation from everyone else.

Variation
You might want to invite people to bring their sheets to a staff meeting and read aloud one or two comments about themselves. If so, encourage people to leave their shyness at the door and allow themselves to share something someone else appreciated about them and feel pride in that accomplishment.

Tips

- Participate. Add your comments to the sheets, too, and make a sheet about you as well. During this kind of activity, act as a team member, not an outsider or boss distanced from the team.
- Give people time to do this, so that they don't leave blank spaces about people and then make some people feel neglected because people had nothing to report next to their name.
- Make this a quarterly happening. It's renewing.

Encourage people to use customer service behaviors in their recognition of each other.

Thanks, I Appreciate That!

This tool encourages staff to publicly thank each other for work well done.

Method

1. Set a few minutes of meeting time during which you invite people to express any thanks to each other that they didn't get a chance to say before.
2. Offer a toast to the group, expressing your admiration and pride. Invite team members to toast one another and the group, identifying people and actions that contributed to service improvement or happy, impressed customers.

Tip

- This can be quick and energizing. Don't drag it out or pull teeth. If people resist, say, "Well, I guess not today!" and move on.

What's Good about Now?

This tool enables your staff to practice the positive in their work and to understand personally what they believe they and others are doing well in the way of service.

Method

1. Comment that the team doesn't stop and talk often enough about what's going well! Ask staff to write nonstop for two minutes on what's good about your service now. The ground rules are as follows:
   —Absolutely nothing negative
   —Even if you're having trouble knowing what to write, don't take your pen off the paper. Keep writing!
2. Give people a minute to censor anything that they don't want to read by circling or crossing it out.
3. Pair people up and ask each person to read what they wrote to that person.
4. Reconvene the group and ask for a few people to volunteer to share their writing with the team.
5. End with the question "How did it feel sharing about this topic?"

Variation:

Rather than doing individual writing, conduct a large group brainstorm and write down anything anyone says to the question "What's good about our service now?"

 ### Tip

- Staff may need a writing warm-up, like "Write nonstop about your day" just to move them from what they were just working on to the topic at hand.

 ## Quick Sentence-Starter Warm-Ups

This tool helps build habitual attention to positive events and service accomplishments in staff meetings.

Method

Start the meeting by asking the group to quickly take a turn completing one of these sentence starters:

- One good thing that happened for me this week at work was . . .
- When I think about our team, I feel good about . . .
- One thing that we're doing well is . . .

- One way people help others here is . . .
- One example of great service we provided this week is . . .
- One thing [a team member] did this week to provide great service to a customer was . . .

Variation

Place one question on each of a few sheets of flipchart paper and have someone (or you) record the answers. Then place the flipcharts in a prominent place for a week so that everyone can see them and feel pride in their work.

Tips

- Invite your team to think of other sentence starters in the same vein.
- Participate yourself. Don't just listen. Act like a full-fledged member of the team.

Tools That Help Staff Appreciate Their Own Service Contributions

Recognition from you and recognition from peers still doesn't cover the subject. Ultimately, people should be able to feel good by patting themselves on the back! You can help them by introducing ways to encourage them to appreciate themselves for their own contributions to impressive service.

Appreciate Me!

Help staff identify their own service skills and accomplishments with this appreciation tool.[1]

Method

1. Before a staff meeting, send out a message asking each team member to write down five service accomplishments from that week that they personally achieved. Give them two categories: interactions with patients and other external customers, and interactions with coworkers or internal customers. Alert them

that they'll be asked to share this information with the rest of the team at the next meeting.

2. Allow 90 minutes for this staff meeting. Explain that you are going to ask each person to share their accomplishments and what they think they do best with the group. Tell them that after each person has talked, there will be an opportunity for three or so people to tell that person what they appreciate about them as well, especially what that person adds to the service team.

3. Take turns focusing on each person and listening to self-appreciation followed by appreciation from the group that will have a reinforcing effect.

Tips

- Your team might have a hard time with this because of self-imposed pressure not to brag, boast, or admit positive things about themselves. Nudge them over this hump. Tell them to abandon any shyness about this and admit what they've accomplished—and that everyone will! While they might be hesitant at first, they're sure to love it.

- Act as the facilitator so you can keep this moving. Just be careful that you don't make people feel cut off while they're sharing.

- Bring this activity back every six months to renew the atmosphere of appreciation surrounding your service. In the meantime, use other tools that accomplish the same purpose.

Success of the Week

This tool has two purposes:[2]

1. To focus people on what's going well in the way of service
2. To make it easy for staff to share their service successes

Method

1. At the start of a staff meeting, ask people to think about a service interaction or incident that they feel pretty good about.

2. Give them a minute to share this interaction or incident with a partner.

3. After a couple of minutes, ask people to share with the larger group what their partner did. If it's a large group, invite a few sample stories. If it's a small group, invite everyone to share their partner's story.
4. Ask people which story they would like to select as service success of the week. Try to reach consensus.
5. Ask someone to volunteer to write up the success of the week and post it on a bulletin board along with a Polaroid of the person sharing the story.

Variations
Alternate the focus, for instance talk about the following:

- A success with a customer
- A success with an internal customer
- A success in maintaining composure while serving a customer

Tips

- This method picks up momentum as people get a bit competitive. Consider this competition healthy, since it's related to service improvement.
- Don't complicate this technique by developing criteria for selecting the success of the week. Keep it simple and straightforward.

The Nicest Compliment

This tool will help your staff admit service successes to the group.[3]

Method

1. At the beginning of a staff meeting, ask staff to think about a compliment they received from a customer.
2. Go around the room letting everyone share a compliment story, including a description of the incident and how it made them feel.
3. Process the activity by asking for common themes and how people felt being thanked.
4. Make this point: We all need to feel needed and appreciated for the service we provide. It feels good when we hear that we're meeting or exceeding our customers' needs.

Tip

- Over time, staff will remember the compliments they receive more often and participation will go up. At first, people might not be attuned to remember the compliments, just the complaints! That's the hidden agenda here—to help staff tune into and remember the positive things their customers say about them.

What I Like about My Job

Help staff share what they like about their service roles with this tool.[4]

Method

1. Ask staff to write down the things that they like about their work with customers, including specific tasks like taking a history, or more global aspects of the job, like solving customer complaints.
2. Give the group 10 to 15 minutes to complete the task, including a few minutes in which to share their list with another person in the group.
3. Ask pairs to call out the kinds of things on their lists and capture these on flipcharts.
4. Ask the group to review their own lists and rank order the items based on the following:
   —Things they like doing
   —Things they think they do well
5. Ask them then to consider the following:
   —What do you like about the items you chose?
   —Was there a relationship between the ones you enjoy doing and the ones you do well?
   —What activities do we all seem to enjoy?
   —What activities are low on many of our lists?

Tips

- As if you didn't know already, participate! Share about yourself, too.

- Don't force people to draw conclusions. Just ask questions that invite them to do so. The real goal is to talk about the activities and responsibilities people enjoy and are good at, and to learn about the people in the process.

Self-Thoughts

This tool is intended as a way to record thoughts that you are having and to find a process of self-encouragement.

Method
Teach this process to your staff:

1. Twice a week take three minutes to write nonstop on your self-thoughts. For example, "I'm thinking that I can't take on one more project. I feel overloaded, and it makes me feel like I'm not good at what I do. I want to feel appreciated and want to know that people think I do a good job."
2. Circle any self-thoughts that are negative.
3. Take another three minutes, examining one negative self-thought and writing about how you might change that thought:
   —I want to feel appreciated. I'm going to start appreciating myself more by changing my attitude about not getting appreciation.
   —I'm going to take out the thank-you notes that people have written and read them when I feel unappreciated.
   —I'm going to do something for someone else and appreciate myself for it.
   —When someone recognizes me for my work, I'm not going to brush it off. I'm going to take in the compliment and really allow myself to feel it.
4. Reread your journal from time to time and appreciate your progress.

Tip

- Challenge people to try this for a month diligently, by which time it will become a habit. People will also be able to see progress in their thinking.

Daily Self-Acknowledgment

This tool helps staff to acknowledge themselves daily for their accomplishments.

Method

Suggest this exercise to your staff or find someone experimental who will try it and then teach it.

1. Before you fall into bed, take about five minutes for yourself, and do the following:
   —Acknowledge yourself for what you have accomplished that day.
   —Acknowledge the qualities that make up who you are.
   —Think about and appreciate the love and care you have given that day and the love and care you have received.

Tip

- At first, it helps to write down your thoughts. Later, these three steps can be done just with closed eyes, deep breathing, and relaxation.

Tools That Help Customers Give Positive Feedback Directly to Staff

This kind of appreciation cannot be the staple food of your service, because it's inappropriate to press customers to give staff feedback if they aren't inclined to. But, many enjoy giving staff feedback, and not just negative feedback, if you make it easy for them to do so.

Patient Satisfaction Recognition

This tool recognizes employees whose behavior has contributed to patient and family satisfaction, as reported by patients and families.

Method

If you receive or become aware of any complimentary letters from patients, their families, or other members of the public, the following are ways to make sure employees receive the recognition they deserve:

1. Read the letters in staff meetings.
2. Reference letters in the comments section of the employee per-formance review.
3. Post employees' pictures and letters where others can see them, for example, on bulletin boards, in display cases, in the lunch room or cafeteria, and the like.
4. Send a copy of the letter to the administrator in charge of your facility and let the employee know you've done this.
5. Invite the patient/family member in to tell their story of how the employee helped them at a staff meeting.
6. Create a big display in the hallway with caricatures of fish hanging from fishing poles and a washtub as a pond. Above it, hang the sign "Fishing for Compliments." Patients will be amused and stop to throw compliments in the pond. Then, have some-one read the fish at each staff meeting.
7. Send a thank-you letter about the customer compliment to the employee at home where they're likely to show it to their family.

Tip

• Invite staff ideas about how to get patient and customer compli-ments, too. They might show some creativity that you're too mild-mannered to display.

Appreciation Cards and Posters

This tool provides a way that patients, families, and others can appreciate staff for impressive customer service.

Method

1. Create an appreciation card that can be filled out by a patient, family member, or community member to let staff know about a job well done.
2. In order for your external customers to know that this is impor-tant to you, create a poster and hang it next to a bin with the appreciation cards. The poster should encourage your cus-tomers to let staff know how well they're doing.

3. Pass on appreciation to staff whenever you receive it from customers and in whatever form:

To: Meg Fonner

From: Joe Herron

Re: Compliment by Patient

A patient to our practice, Gail Potter, called today to inform me she was very impressed with the warm, good-natured, informative response you gave her recently when she inquired about a confusing bill we sent her.

Her call was most uplifting to me, and I am only too happy to relate her comments to you. As the call progressed, my thoughts turned to our customer service commitment and how you exemplify this commitment in the way you treat your customers.

I thanked her for sharing her positive feeling and assured her I would inform you of her call.

Congratulations!

Tips

- To enhance this process, let your customers in on your customer service behaviors and standards by listing them on the back of the appreciation card and having a place on the card to list the number of the relevant behavior or standard that they saw or experienced.
- Build in a special bonus for staff members whom customers recognize for your behavior of the month/quarter.

Bell-Ringing Celebration

This tool has two main purposes:

1. To encourage staff to pay attention to patient satisfaction results and to have targets
2. To recognize staff when they accomplish the goal or target

Method

1. When you hear of a positive result, a problem solved, or satisfied customers, ring a bell and have employees convene for a two-minute *Ta-daah!*
2. Provide candy kisses, popcorn, or sodas.

 Tips

- Try to surprise employees.
- If you have more then one shift, make sure that everyone gets equal attention.

 ## Banner Appreciation

Make public any positive customer results with banners and other visible signs.

Method

Show positive results on a banner (for example, "Ta-daah! In October 95 percent of our customers were highly satisfied when we _____).

 Tip

- Make a big deal about hanging the banner. Encourage as many staff as possible to be there and celebrate!

General Tips for Recognizing Staff

- Use a mix of methods since staff get bored of any method done too often without variety.
- The methods need to focus on specific behavior, not global or general compliments. They need to specify what exactly the staff member did that contributed to customer satisfaction.
- Ideally, you will not be the sole dispenser of recognition. Instead, you will set up methods that enable positive feedback to flow from staff to staff and from customers to staff. And hopefully, you will also help staff build the self-appreciation skills that enable them to

carry around in their heads and hearts words of appreciation for their own generous service to customers.

Conclusion

This chapter addressed maintaining your service focus. Imagine letting all of your hard work fade because an "out of sight, out of mind" mentality takes over. **Hold tight** to your service focus. Pay attention to service **every day, or it** withers away as a priority in people's minds. **Gradually, as you persist** in your attention to service, you will create a **current in your** service that carries people along toward higher performance and heightened customer satisfaction.

Notes

1. Adapted, with permission, from Gail Scott & Associates © 1997.

2. Ibid.

3. Ibid.

4. Ibid.

Chapter 8

• • •

Getting Personal

This book includes a multitude of tools to support seven basic service strategies. These strategies aren't linear. You don't have to use first one, then another, then another in order to get results. You might decide to start with just one strategy and go deep with it. Or develop a three-strategy approach, starting with one strategy first, then later a second, and later a third. Or you can pick the big three strategies and start small efforts related to each all at once. Remember this:

- There is no best approach.
- There is no best sequence.

Not Sure Where to Start?

Where should you start? Look back at the start of each chapter. There are questions that help you to determine whether each strategy can produce benefits for your service. Revisit those and list the strategies that fit your needs.

Ask yourself if you can do more than one at a time since different people might be involved. For instance, if you have staff members involved in the hiring process, they might start using the tools provided to hire service savvy people. At the same time, marketing people or others good at group facilitation could launch some voice-of-the-customer tools. If different people do different work, you can accomplish more than one strategy at a time. If all staff need to be somehow involved, its better to pick and choose so as not to overload your people and circuits.

So what's the best way to choose?

1. List the strategies that you want to consider because they all would be good for your service and team.
2. Talk with others and determine whether your service needs a natural or logical sequence to these strategies.
3. If there is no best sequence from your team's viewpoint, develop criteria for choosing among the strategies that compete for your attention. Then, evaluate the alternatives using the criteria. Here's an example using the CQI tool called the decision matrix. In the left-hand column are alternative strategies that address your service needs. Across the top are criteria for evaluating these alternatives. Get a team of staff together.
   —Agree on which criteria the group wants to use to select among possible strategies.
   —Have each individual rate the alternatives using the criteria.
   —Have people tally their scores across for each alternative.
   —Make a grand chart in which you add together everyone's scores for alternative 1, 2, 3, and so on.
   —See which strategies win. Discuss people's comfort level with pursuing the winner. Talk it through until you agree on how to proceed.

Here's an example: If you need *all* of the seven strategies, your decision matrix might look like this:

Decision Matrix

Key: (1 = low, 3 = high)				
Strategy	Potential Impact	Likelihood of Staff Support	Easy, Doable	Total
Hiring for service				
Voice of customer				
Set service standards				
Remove service barriers				
Reduce customer anxiety				
Help staff deal in high-stress environment				
Maintain service focus				

The key thing to remember is that the strategies included here don't have stopping points. They need to be ongoing, although the tools you use to support each strategy can stop, start, and vary.

For instance, consider the strategy "Help Staff Hear the Voices of Their Customers." This needs to be done continually, but some of the ways you choose to do this might have beginnings and endings. Let's say you decide to institute a regular ongoing system of monthly focus groups with former patients. You can do these month after month and get very valuable feedback and advice from patients. The focus group tool can be ongoing. Or, you can periodically change approaches and use another tool, "Staff as Pulse Takers," with customers instead of or in addition to additional approaches. Helping staff hear the voices of their customers needs to be enduring, but you can vary the tools for accomplishing this.

For the strategy "Hire Service Savvy People," you will at some point start up practices that accomplish this, and you will continue using those practices. And how about the strategy "Remove Barriers"? Up front, you might tackle several barriers in a row and really chase after them. Because barriers to delivering impressive service come and go, and new ones emerge, barrier removal is something you need to do continuously.

So, we hope you adopt the strategies as ongoing strategies to achieve impressive service, selecting tools now and then as needed to support and renew these strategies, giving them staying power.

You Don't Have to Do This Alone

Not only don't you have to do this alone, you can't do this alone. And you shouldn't. One positive consequence of the turbulence in health care today is that people are realizing that working together and supporting one another are essential to delivering quality care and service to patients. None of us can do this alone. The silos are slowly beginning to crumble as we come to realize how we need each other to pool resources and energy for the good of our patients and other customers.

Structures That Build Support

Many organizations are doing great things to build interdependence and support teamwork. As a result, many managers are realizing the following for the first time:

- I don't have to have all of the answers. I can learn from other people's experience.
- I don't have to own all of the resources. We can share tools, techniques, and even people.
- I don't have to feel isolated. There are others in this with me, thinking and feeling the way I do.

Manager Support Groups

Consider building support for yourself! Reinstitute one of those brown bag lunch clubs for yourself and other managers. Spend time together bouncing ideas around, informally tackling problems, and checking in on how each of you feels about changes and plans.

Or try forming a more formal manager support group or mentor team. Form small teams of managers that get together to provide peer coaching, networking, and support. The idea is to create a balance and mix of ideas, perspectives, and disciplines. Knowing that most of us are inclined to go to the people we know and trust for help and support, we tend to miss out on the great benefits of interacting with managers in different realms and with different perspectives. For those trying to create seamless systems, we need to expand our networks. The people who don't see things exactly as you do can open your eyes to other ways of seeing your services and the possibilities for enhancing them.

Are you thinking, "Sounds good, but who has the time or energy to put this kind of thing together?" Consider these examples:

- Amy Unrath at Saint Mary's Hospital in Green Bay, Wisconsin, has been helping her managers work together and learn from each other very successfully for more than six years with very positive results, all with the goal of supporting the service improvement initiative. Amy trained several leaders to act as facilitators or coaches of small manager support groups. These leaders facilitated and scheduled meetings, and they also got together to pool lessons and set the future direction for the groups.

• Steve Mandle and Pam Fink formed a team at Parkland Hospital and Health System in Dallas, Texas, that uses several techniques to support managers in their service improvement journey. Their department alignment committee consists of leaders representing all of the organization's different entities. This team's charge is to make sure that the different entities are all involved in the system's theme-of-the-quarter campaigns (similar to the one-behavior-at-a-time approach in chapter 7). Committee members share ideas and techniques that are being used and developed by their managers, so that other people can apply successful strategies within their own areas. Members of the education department facilitate the committee and also publish a wonderful service improvement newsletter that shares ideas and updates with their 6,000 employees. (For information contact Steve Mandle or Pam Fink at Education Department, Dallas County Hospital Dist./Parkland, 5201 Harry Hines Blvd., Dallas, Texas 75235.)

Such strategies keep managers connected to each other and enable them to learn from one another. Also, as people tend to do related things, they provide the glue that holds together different work teams and managers.

Support for Staff

Although there are great benefits to meeting with other managers to compare notes and learn from each other, don't stop there. Solidify the spirit of partnership with your staff and multiply the support for you and your team by considering another approach to support, namely development of a service representative program. Every manager chooses a representative from his or her area to be trained as a service representative. Service reps receive training in facilitation skills, communication, and problem solving.

Reps meet monthly to discuss developments throughout the system and in other teams in pursuit of impressive service. They learn new tools that help solve service problems and handle complaints with effective service recovery. They generate ideas that enhance the individual team initiatives, and then meet with their managers to share what they've learned. Together the manager and the service rep plan a monthly skill-building meeting or update related to service for the rest of their team.

These duos are powerful! The folks at Maine General Health System in Augusta and Waterville, Maine, have been using a service rep system like this for several years and agree that the ideas, enthusiasm, and involvement of frontline employees are what keep service initiatives alive and kicking. At Maine General, the service representatives also plan events designed to recognize and celebrate service improvement. (For information, contact Lorette Cromett at Education & Organization Development, Maine General Health, 6 East Chestnut Street, Augusta, Maine 04330-9988.)

Consider these and other ways to develop support for yourself and other managers in your organization so that you all work together and learn from each other in pursuit of impressive service. The result is collective strength!

But what if you're working in an organization that doesn't share your vision? What if there is no organizational commitment to service improvement, or at least no commitment as visible as those in the above examples? You can still develop support for yourself.

Return to the brown bag lunch idea. Gather a few other leaders to work together on service improvement. Give your friends a copy of this book. Divide up some of the tools and plan to get together to share experiences and results.

Meet with the other members of your organization and plan a way for several managers to do this together. Consider the support group and service rep concepts. Or form a service improvement committee made up of frontline staff from several departments or services.

Positive energy has to start somewhere, and it can start with you! Although there are certainly payoffs if you are working in a system that has made a large commitment to improving service, you shouldn't feel that you have to do this alone no matter where you work.

Don't Keep Your Learning Private

- Keep notes. Document your journey. Better yet, write it up so that others can learn from you.
- Involve your staff and prepare a presentation at a leadership meeting. Share your story. You'll help others and boost your own energy.

- Take staff on the road. Let them present the story at a local or national conference. You will expand your own professional network that way and find other like-minded souls for strategy swapping.

In short, the turtle only moves forward when it sticks its neck out. Stick your neck out. Take the initiative to start up a service improvement support system for yourself and others. Most people have something to share and want to share it, and all can learn and become bolder in the process.

Do You Have What It Takes?

You have an *interest* in achieving impressive service or you wouldn't have read this far. And now you have even more *tools* to help advance impressive service within your team. That's a help, but it's not enough.

In a quiet, personal moment, ask yourself the following:

- Am I convinced that the payoffs of improving service are worth the sweat it takes, or are mixed feelings causing me to waver? Am I sold on the belief that impressive service is worth the chase?
- Can I *picture* impressive service in all its richness? Can I see it in my mind's eye? Can I see, taste, smell, hear, and touch it?
- Can I communicate my vision of impressive service to my team? Can I put it in words? Can I help others see it?
- Can I telegraph my *commitment*? Can I convey a genuine passion for achieving impressive service? Can I show that the very idea of it *moves* me?
- Do I have the personal discipline to *focus* on service when so many pressures compete for my attention?

The pursuit of impressive service is an ambitious undertaking. Fortunately, you can work at it gradually so that it doesn't overwhelm either you or your team. But still, it's an ambitious undertaking because it requires more than an interest and more than a tool kit.

The pursuit of impressive service requires this of you:

- Clarity
- Vision
- Resolve

- Passion
- Focus

Clarity

You have to believe that the results of your efforts to achieve impressive service will be worth the work involved. You need to be clear about this. If you aren't clear about it, then you'll allow competing pressures to push you off course. If you have the slightest doubt in your own clarity about this or any mixed feelings, complete the following worksheet and see where your thinking leads you.

Weighing the Costs and Benefits

Pursuit of impressive service is worth the effort because . . .	Pursuit of impressive service is not really worth the effort because . . .
•	•
•	•
•	•

Now look at the reasons not to pursue impressive service and respond. See if you can talk yourself out of these misgivings. If you can't, your mixed feelings are going to interfere with your role as champion of service improvement, and your mixed feelings will show.

Vision

If you're a believer in the importance of moving forward to pursue impressive service, that's great—but it's not enough. You need a vision of what impressive service looks like. You can flesh out elements of a vision by listening to customers and considering what satisfies you when you're wearing a consumer hat. But at some point, you need to crystallize your own personal vision of impressive service—one so compelling that you can see, feel, smell, taste, and touch it. Your vision has to take on a life of its own, driving your energies and focus.

If you want impressive service but don't feel clear about how that would look concretely given the service you manage, walk yourself through these steps and see where it leads you.

1. List each of your key customer groups.
2. For each customer group, imagine you find them raving to friends and neighbors about how wonderful your service was in their recent experience. List the adjectives you wish people in this group would use as they rave.
3. Now, for each adjective, jot down words to describe the *facts* you wish were true about your service—facts that would lead customers to use this adjective.

Your Vision of Impressive Service

Customer Group: _____	
Adjectives You Wish They Used to Describe Your Services	Facts You Wish Were True about Your Service That Would Ensure Use of These Adjectives
•	•
•	•
•	•

Now, in a nutshell, crystallize your vision of impressive service in a few sentences:

My Vision of Impressive Service

If you can't picture it, it's going to be hard to create. Ask for help from customers and staff in developing a powerful service vision so this vision doesn't get cloudy in an atmosphere saturated with other priorities.

Resolve

Determination ... tenacity ... drive—the resolve that stops any naysayers or cynics from running you off course. Inevitably, there will be some staff who say, "How can we possibly do this given everything else?" or "Now what? Yet another priority?" or "This too shall pass! It's just another flash in the pan" or "All well and good, but who can afford this?" These and other words all have the potential of diminishing anything short of unflinching resolve on your part.

Anticipate what members of your staff, family, and colleagues might say to question or pooh-pooh your striving for impressive service. Prepare yourself to respond without changing direction.

How Can I Counteract the Counterforces?

What people might say to push me off course	How I can respond so that I don't lose my way
•	•
•	•
•	•

Passion

You might think we've gone too far with this one. We don't think so. Really effective managers who achieve impressive service attach emotion to their vision and resolve. They really *want* great service with the kind of energy and determination that comes when your heart, not just your head, is propelling you.

Do some soul-searching here. Why do *you* really want impressive service? What do you stand to gain from it? Is there anything about this pursuit that fills you with feeling or lights your fire?

Express Your Commitment

Write a statement that expresses your commitment to pursuing impressive service. Find a way to make your heart, not just your head, do the talking—even if you're a cerebral sort of person!

Your staff will respond to your energy and feeling, as much as to your words. If you lack energy and feeling, theirs will be lackluster, too, as will your service improvement efforts.

Focus

Even if all of the above are in place, *focus* is a necessity and, in today's environment, it's not one bit easy. Picture the Ping-Pong game where your eye follows the ball back and forth. Health care used to be somewhat like a Ping-Pong game—balls flying in predictable directions. But the game has really changed. Many balls are flying simultaneously, and many of them are coming at you faster than you can catch them. Imagine trying to hang on to one Ping-Pong ball and throw it, with good aim, in the midst of this chaos! Its a real challenge. Undoubtedly, in your job, you have multiple priorities and many forces flying at you. Not only is it hard to hold on to any one chosen priority, it's also very hard to propel it in the desired direction when you're so busy reacting to what's flying toward you and following the random flight of balls.

Do you have the self-discipline to hang on tightly to the impressive service ball and, having a good grip on it, send it flying in the desired direction in spite of everything else going on in your environment and commanding your attention?

Conclusion

Recently, an administrator said to one of the authors, "We really want to improve customer service, but people are overloaded and overwhelmed. We have to figure out how to improve customer service in a way that is not complex. It has to be a simple way." The author answered, "There is only one *simple* way to improve customer service and that is this: Managers have to pay attention to it!"

You're probably thinking, "What's simple about that?" It is simple. It just isn't easy. This book is full of tools you can use if you pay attention to service. Any one of these tools leads you in the right direction. You don't have to use all of them, and you don't even have to use genius in sequencing your efforts. You need to start somewhere and keep your attention on service.

Imagine the sculptor. Most sculptors picture a work of art in their mind's eye. Then they get the best tools they can find. And they use those tools to chip away at the material until they eventually create the work of art. If they're using hard rock or resistant material, this is a slow, tedious process—but with vision, resolve, the right tools, and passion, they will create that work of art.

So it is with impressive service. If you develop and apply clarity, vision, resolve, passion, and focus, you can also create the work of art that is impressive service.

Index